Qui...

Child Sexual Exploitation

*For Healthcare, Social Services,
and Law Enforcement Professionals*

G.W. Medical Publishing, Inc.
St. Louis
www.gwmedical.com

CONTENTS IN BRIEF

Quick Reference
Child Sexual Exploitation

*For Healthcare, Social Services,
and Law Enforcement Professionals*

Sharon W. Cooper, MD, FAAP
Adjunct Associate Professor of Pediatrics
University of North Carolina School
of Medicine
Chapel Hill, North Carolina
Clinical Assistant Professor of Pediatrics
Uniformed Services University of
Health Sciences
Bethesda, Maryland
Chief, Developmental & Forensic Pediatric
Service, Womack Army Medical Center
Fort Bragg, North Carolina
Instructor, National Center for Missing &
Exploited Children
Alexandria, Virginia

Richard J. Estes, DSW, ACSW
Professor
Chair, Concentration in Social and
Economic Development
Director, International Programs
University of Pennsylvania School of
Social Work
Philadelphia, Pennsylvania

Angelo P. Giardino, MD, PhD, MPH, FAAP
Medical Director
Texas Children's Health Plan
Associate Clinical Professor of Pediatrics
Baylor College of Medicine
Attending Physician
Children's Assessment Center
Texas Children's Hospital
Houston, Texas

Nancy D. Kellogg, MD
Professor of Pediatrics
University of Texas Health Science Center at
San Antonio
Medical Director
Childsafe
Medical Director
Christus Santa Rosa Center for Miracles

Victor I. Vieth, JD
Director
NDAA's Child Abuse Programs
National Child Protection Training Center
Winona State University
Winona, Minnesota

G.W. Medical Publishing, Inc.
St. Louis
www.gwmedical.com

Publishers: Glenn E. Whaley and Marianne V. Whaley
Art Director: Glenn E. Whaley
Managing Editors: Karen C. Maurer
                  Megan O. Hayes
Associate Editors: Robert J. Lewis
                   Christine M. Bauer
Book Design/Page Layout: G.W. Graphics
                         Sudon Choe
                         Charles J. Seibel, III
Print/Production Coordinator: Charles J. Seibel, III
Cover Design: G.W. Graphics
Color Prepress Specialist: Charles J. Seibel, III
Developmental Editor: Elaine Steinborn
Copy Editor: Sheri Kubasek
Indexer: Robert A. Saigh

Printed in Canada

Publisher:
G.W. Medical Publishing, Inc.
77 Westport Plaza, Suite 366, St. Louis, Missouri 63146-3124 USA
Phone: (314)542-4213 Fax: (314)542-4239 Toll Free: (800)600-0330
http://www.gwmedical.com

Library of Congress Cataloging-in-Publication Data

Child sexual exploitation quick reference : for healthcare, social service, and law enforcement.
    p. cm.
  By Sharon Cooper ... [et al.]
  ISBN 1-878060-21-X (alk. paper)
  1. Child sexual abuse. 2. Child sexual abuse--United States. 3. Children--Crimes against.
  4. Children--Crimes against--United States. I. Cooper, Sharon, 1952-
  HV6570.C58 2006
  362.76--dc22
                        2006029480

CONTRIBUTORS

Mary P. Alexander, MA, LPC
MA Counseling-Marriage and Family Therapy
MEd Educational Psychology and Special
Education
Certified School Counselor
Eagle Nest, New Mexico

Elena Azaola, PhD
PhD in Social Anthropology
Psychoanalyst
Professor at the Center for Advanced Studies
and Research in Social Anthropology
Mexico City, Mexico

Joseph S. Bova Conti, BA
Detective Sergeant, Maryland Heights
Police Department
Crimes Against Children Specialist
Certified Juvenile Specialist — State of
Missouri
Member MPJOA, MJJA, SLCJJA
Lecturer, Author, Consultant
Maryland Heights, Missouri

Duncan T. Brown, Esq
Assistant District Attorney
Sex Crimes/Special Victims Bureau
Richmond County District Attorney's Office
Staten Island, New York

Cormac Callanan, BA, MSc
Secretary General
Association of Internet Hotline Providers in
Europe (INHOPE)
Goring, United Kingdom

Lt. William D. Carson, MA, SPSC
Commander, Bureau of Investigation
Maryland Heights Police Department
Maryland Heights, Missouri

Michelle K. Collins, MA
Director, Exploited Child Unit
National Center for Missing & Exploited
Children (NCMEC)
Alexandria, Virginia

Peter I. Collins, MCA, MD, FRCP(C)
Manager, Forensic Psychiatry Unit
Behavioural Sciences Section
Ontario Provincial Police
Associate Professor, Department of Psychiatry
University of Toronto
Toronto, Ontario, Canada

Jeffrey A. Dort, JD
Deputy District Attorney
Team Leader Family Protection Division
Lead Prosecutor — ICAC: Internet Crimes
Against Children
San Diego District Attorney's Office
San Diego, California

V. Denise Everett, MD, FAAP
Director, Child Sexual Abuse Team
WakeMed
Raleigh, North Carolina
Clinical Associate Professor, Department
of Pediatrics
University of North Carolina at Chapel Hill
School of Medicine
Chapel Hill, North Carolina

Fadi Barakat Fadel
Director of Programmes of the International
Centre to Combat Exploitation of Children
Founder of Sexually Exploited Youth Speak
Out Network (SEYSO)
Victoria, British Columbia, Canada

James A. H. Farrow, MD, FSAM
Professor, Medicine & Pediatrics
Director, Student Health Services
Tulane University
New Orleans, Louisiana

David Finkelhor, PhD
Director, Crimes Against Children
Research Center
Family Research Laboratory
Professor, Department of Sociology
University of New Hampshire
Durham, New Hampshire

Katherine A. Free, MA
Program Manager
Exploited Child Unit
National Center for Missing & Exploited
Children (NCMEC)
Alexandria, Virginia

Nadine Grant
Director of Programs
Save the Children Canada
Toronto, Ontario, Canada

Ernestine S. Gray, JD
Judge
Orleans Parish Juvenile Court
Section "A"
New Orleans, Louisiana

Donald B. Henley
Senior Special Agent
US Department of Homeland Security
Immigration and Customs Enforcement (ICE)
San Francisco, California

Marcia E. Herman-Giddens, PA, DrPH
Child Maltreatment Consulting
Senior Fellow, North Carolina Child
Advocacy Institute
Adjunct Professor, University of North Carolina
School of Public Health
Pittsboro, North Carolina

Nicole G. Ives, MSW
Doctoral Candidate
University of Pennsylvania, School of
Social Work
Philadelphia, Pennsylvania

Eileen R. Jacob
Supervisor Special Agent
Crimes Against Children Unit
Federal Bureau of Investigation
Washington, DC

Terry Jones, BA (Hons), PGCE
Consultant: Internet Paedophilia Training
Awareness Consultancy (IPTAC)
Former Head Greater Manchester Police
Abusive Images Unit
United Kingdom

Aaron Kipnis, PhD
Professor — Clinical Psychology
Pacifica Graduate Institute
Carpenteria, California
Psychologist
Santa Barbara, California

Susan S. Kreston, JD, LLM
Consultant
New Orleans, Louisiana

Kenneth V. Lanning, MS
(Retired FBI)
CAC Consultants
Fredericksburg, Virginia

Mary Anne Layden, PhD
Codirector
Sexual Trauma and Psychopathology Program
Director of Education
Center for Cognitive Therapy
Department of Psychiatry
University of Pennsylvania
Philadelphia, Pennsylvania

Shyla R. Lefever, PhD
Assistant Professor of Communication
Hampton University
Hampton, Virginia

Ingrid Leth
Former Senior Adviser
UNICEF HQ, USA
Associate Professor — Clinical Child
Psychology
Department of Psychology
University of Copenhagen
Copenhagen, Denmark

Elizabeth J. Letourneau, PhD
Assistant Professor
Department of Psychiatry and
Behavioral Sciences
Medical University of South Carolina
Charleston, South Carolina

L. Alvin Malesky, Jr, PhD
Assistant Professor, Department of Psychology
Western Carolina University
Cullowhee, North Carolina

Bernadette McMenamin, AO
National Director of CHILD WISE
ECPAT in Australia
Director, NetAlert (Internet safety advisory board)
Director, KidsAP (Internet safety advisory board)
Advisor to the Federal Government for the
National Plan of Action on CSEC
(Commercial Sexual Exploitation of Children)
South Melbourne, Australia

Kimberly Mitchell, PhD
Research Associate — Crimes Against Children
Research Center
Assistant Research Professor of Psychology
University of New Hampshire
Durham, New Hampshire

Thomas P. O'Connor, BA, MA
Chief of Police, Maryland Heights Police
Department
Law Enforcement Instructor, Specialty Crimes
Against Persons, Criminal Investigation
Procedures
Maryland Heights, Missouri

John Patzakis, Esq
Vice Chairman and Chief Legal Officer
Guidance Software, Inc.
Pasadena, California

David S. Prescott, LICSW
Treatment Assessment Director, Sand Ridge
Secure Treatment Center
Mauston, Wisconsin

Ethel Quayle, BA, MSc, PsychD
Lecturer
Researcher with the COPINE Project
Department of Applied Psychology
University College Cork
Cork, Ireland

Erika Rivera Ragland, JD
Staff Attorney
National Center for Prosecution of Child Abuse
American Prosecutors Research Institute (APRI)
Alexandria, Virginia

Thomas Rickert
Attorney at Law
President, Association of Internet Hotline
Providers in Europe (INHOPE)
Chair, Internet Content Task Force eco
Cologne, Germany

Migael Scherer
Director, Dart Award for Excellence in
Reporting on Victims of Violence
Dart Center for Journalism and Trauma
Department of Communication
University of Washington
Seattle, Washington

Daniel J. Sheridan, PhD, RN, FAAN
Assistant Professor
Johns Hopkins University School of Nursing
President, International Association
of Forensic Nurses
Baltimore, Maryland

Linnea W. Smith, MD
Psychiatrist
Chapel Hill, North Carolina

Raymond C. Smith
Assistant Inspector in Charge
Fraud, Prohibited Mailings and Asset Forfeiture
US Postal Inspection Service
Washington, DC

Max Taylor, PhD, C. Forensic Psychology
Professor and Head of Department
of Applied Psychology
University College Cork
Director, COPINE Project
Cork, Ireland

Govind Prasad Thapa, MA, BL, MPA, PhD
Additional Inspector General, Nepal Police
Chief — Crime Investigation Department
Police Headquarters
Kathmandu, Nepal

Phyllis L. Thompson, LCSW
OUR KIDS Center
Nashville General Hospital
Instructor in the Department of Pediatrics
Vanderbilt University Medical Center
Nashville, Tennessee

Christopher D. Trifiletti
Special Agent
Federal Bureau of Investigation
Baltimore, Maryland
Chair, Interpol Specialists Group on Crimes
Against Children, Child Pornography, and
Internet Investigations Theme Groups
Lyon, France

Dawn Van Pelt, BSN, RN
Graduate Student
Johns Hopkins University School of Nursing
Baltimore, Maryland

Bharathi A. Venkatraman, Esq
United States Department of Justice
Civil Rights Division
Washington, DC

F. Bruce Watkins, MD
Assistant Clinical Professor of Ob/Gyn
University of Illinois College of Medicine
Medical Director, Women's Health Service
Crusader Clinic
Rockford, Illinois

Bruce Watson, LLB, CA
Past President, Enough Is Enough
Fairfax, Virginia

Neil Alan Weiner, PhD
Senior Research Investigator
Center for Research on Youth and Social Policy
School of Social Work
University of Pennsylvania
Philadelphia, Pennsylvania

Cathy Spatz Widom, PhD
Professor of Psychiatry and University Professor
UMDNJ — New Jersey Medical School
Department of Psychiatry
Newark, New Jersey

Janis Wolak, JD
Research Assistant Professor
Crimes Against Children Research Center
University of New Hampshire
Durham, New Hampshire

FOREWORD

In my career as a prosecutor, and now as a congressman, I have seen tremendous improvements in our nation's response to cases of child maltreatment. In most communities today, multidisciplinary teams work together for the best interests of children. Many elected district attorneys, sheriffs, and police chiefs have developed specialized units to respond to cases of child abuse.

Perhaps the most important development is the Children's Advocacy Center program. Children's Advocacy Centers (CACs) are child-friendly facilities where children can be interviewed sensitively and receive medical and psychological services. As a district attorney, I had the privilege of starting the nation's first CAC. As a member of Congress, I championed support for my National Children's Advocacy Center in Huntsville, Alabama, and also for the National Children's Alliance, a coalition of CACs from across the nation that is head-quartered in Washington, DC. Today there are hundreds of CACs in every part of our country.

Through the work of many organizations and training centers, thousands of frontline professionals are trained annually in the art and science of handling child protection cases. In the specific area of child sexual exploitation, this quick reference will provide them a wealth of information that can be accessed from any location.

We cannot, however, rest on our laurels. Commercial exploitation of children is a global problem that impacts every community in the United States, and there is some evidence to suggest that these children are just as likely to come from rural and suburban communities as urban centers. Additionally, modern technology poses a new threat to our children. It is increasingly easy for perpetrators to exploit children through the Internet, to create and disseminate child pornography, and to solicit children for illicit purposes.

I want to commend the frontline investigators, prosecutors, medical and mental health professionals, and other child advocates who are in the trenches daily trying to spare children from every form of exploitation. It is for them that this book is written. You labor long hours for little pay or honor on behalf of someone else's children. Please know that your selfless dedication is not unnoticed. Indeed, your heroism is an inspiration to us all.

Congressman Robert E. "Bud" Cramer, Jr.
Member of the US House of Representatives (1999-present)
Founder of the Children's Advocacy Center movement

FOREWORD

It is common to hear pronouncements from public figures that children are society's most important and treasured assets. To an overwhelming majority, this concept is fundamentally true. To a marginal and deviant minority, however, children are viewed as a commodity to be traded, imported, and exported like any other piece of merchandise. Parents and professionals need help combating the alarming growth of child exploitation, and this book is a valuable tool in the fight to protect our children from predators who would use them for financial gain or prurient reasons.

The information in *Child Sexual Exploitation Quick Reference* was contributed by individuals who represent a wide array of backgrounds, disciplines, and perspectives. Some speak from distant lands that are growing ever closer with the ease of air travel and where youths are being sold to travelers seeking to indulge their perverse needs with someone else's children. Some voices are actually electronic particles from cyberspace delivering images of unspeakable abuse to our home and office computers.

The 2-volume set from which this quick reference is derived is the most comprehensive text on this subject that I have seen, and it represents the efforts of an impressive collection of premier investigators, judicial participants, child protection agency personnel, and clinicians. This quick reference maintains the same quality of research and is invaluable for frontline professionals who deal with the victims and perpetrators of child sexual exploitation.

Robert M. Reece, MD

Clinical Professor of Pediatrics
Tufts University School of Medicine
Visiting Professor of Pediatrics
Dartmouth Medical School
Editor, *The Quarterly Update*

PREFACE

When the concept of mass communication began with Gutenberg's printing press in the 14th century, its purpose was to disperse information and promote new ideas. Seven centuries later, the Internet has expanded upon the original purpose of the printing press and now threatens the deception and entrapment of our most vulnerable resource: children. As methods of victimization have become more innovative, sophisticated, and elusive, professionals are challenged in their efforts to prevent, detect, intervene, and treat children that fall victim to online predators.

Knowledge of Internet crimes against children has been primarily limited to media coverage of the topic. This text serves to separate fact from fiction and to dispel several myths and misconceptions, including the belief that prostituted youths typically market themselves by choice and can easily escape from this form of abuse. To the uninformed, it is inconceivable that children and youths are often sold from within their own homes, that the Internet is used in numerous capacities to make such arrangements, and that Internet cafés present a nearly untraceable means of making the deal. Online solicitation has become an increasing threat to children. Many naïve children and youths unwittingly receive unwanted sexual solicitations and may be enticed to leave their homes and families to meet online predators; such encounters may end tragically in sexual or physical assault, abduction, or murder. Images of abuse can now be taken and disseminated with Web cameras, mobile/cellular phones, and video iPods. What was slavery and bondage in the past has now become human trafficking for forced labor and sexual exploitation. These crimes continue to escalate worldwide.

Investigations of high profile cases of sexual exploitation have resulted in an organized response to sex tourists, child pornographers, and pimps of prostituted children. Guidelines on how to identify and respond to sexual exploitation situations are listed clearly in this quick reference for law enforcement, medical, and social science professionals who work with victims and offenders directly.

From a child maltreatment perspective, this groundbreaking work provides comprehensive and diverse information on this contemporary, yet daunting and misunderstood, form of child abuse. As the Internet, the "printing press" of the 21st century, has opened new doors for the worldwide exchange of information and ideas, so too has it opened a Pandora's box of opportunities for criminals who victimize children and youths. At present, the knowledge of Internet crimes against children is fragmented, scant, and discipline specific. This text is a step toward comprehension, effective intervention, and the multidisciplinary coordination of frontline investigations of crimes involving exploited children. It will open your eyes and your mind to a new dark side of child abuse that we can no longer afford to ignore.

Sharon W. Cooper, MD, FAAP
Richard J. Estes, DSW, ACSW
Angelo P. Giardino, MD, PhD, MPH, FAAP
Nancy D. Kellogg, MD
Victor I. Vieth, JD

CONTENTS IN DETAIL

CHAPTER 12: LEGAL ISSUES SPECIFIC TO PORNOGRAPHY CASES

CHAPTER 13: LEGAL CONSIDERATIONS IN PROSTITUTION CASES

Quick Reference

Child Sexual Exploitation

*For Healthcare, Social Services,
and Law Enforcement Professionals*

G.W. Medical Publishing, Inc.
St. Louis
www.gwmedical.com

Chapter 1

OVERVIEW

Sharon W. Cooper, MD, FAAP
Richard J. Estes, DSW, ACSW
V. Denise Everett, MD, FAAP
Marcia E. Herman-Giddens, PA, DrPH
Aaron Kipnis, PhD
Mary Anne Layden, PhD
Ingrid Leth, Former Senior Adviser, UNICEF
Linnea W. Smith, MD
Neil Alan Weiner, PhD

PHYSICAL ABUSE

— Reports of child abuse and neglect in the United States have risen steadily (Sedlak & Broadhurst, 1996) and have doubled in the latter half of the 1990s.

— Over 1 million children suffer moderate injuries each year; about 160 000 are severely injured; and over 1000 die from parental abuse or neglect.

— 1 in 50 US children is physically abused (US Dept of Health & Human Services [USDHHS], 1993).

— Almost 80% of perpetrators are parents; other relatives account for an additional 10%.

— The average age of abused children is 7 years; the average age of abusers is 31 years.

— Most of the children who are murdered, seriously injured, physically abused, or medically neglected are boys, especially boys with disabilities (Sobsey et al, 1997).

— Rates of maltreatment:

1. Are lowest among children who live with both biological parents (Blankenhorn, 1995).

2. Are slightly higher when divorced fathers have custody.

3. Are highest among children with single mothers, particularly when a nonbiological man lives in the house (Margolin, 1992).

4. Are almost 7 times higher among children whose families have an annual income less than $15 000, compared to children whose families have greater income levels.

5. Reflect greatest statistical risk of abuse or neglect for boys of single mothers who have young children and are living below poverty level as well as children of alcoholic and drug-addicted parents of both genders (Horn, 1998).

— Results of abuse:

1. Victims can experience academic, emotional, and economic failure (Burton et al, 1994).

2. Child victims tend to have early difficulty in school.

3. Abused boys are more likely to drink more, abuse more drugs, and suffer more juvenile arrests at earlier ages than nonabused boys (Cooley-Quille et al, 1995).

4. Abused boys are 3 times more likely to become aggressive and violent (Gilligan, 1996; Smith & Thornberry, 1995).

5. Boys' violence toward abusive caregivers often leads to long-term incarceration.

6. In over 60% of all murders committed by teenaged boys, the victims are adult men or family members who are abusing them (Dawson & Langan, 1994).

7. Boys abused by mothers are more likely to abuse their spouses when adults.

8. Women abused by spouses are more at risk for abusing boys, completing the cycle of violence.

SEXUAL ABUSE

— Sexual involvement among children and adolescents is widespread.

— Most sexually abused children are girls.

— 61% of all high school seniors have had sexual intercourse, about half are currently sexually active, and 21% have had at least 4 partners (Committee on Public Education [CPE], 2001).

— 74% of girls who had intercourse before age 14 years and 60% of those who had intercourse before age 15 years did so involuntarily (CPE, 2001).

— As many as two thirds of teenaged mothers report they were forced to have sex with adult men when they were younger.

— Rape crisis centers document acquaintance and date rape in 70% to 80% of cases.

— The United States has one of the highest teenaged pregnancy rates worldwide.

— Persons younger than 25 years account for two thirds of all cases of sexually transmitted diseases (STDs) (CPE, 2001), and there are 12 million new cases annually (Brownback, 2001).

SOCIAL INFLUENCES

— Although Western societies generally consider it perverted for adults to have sex with children, other societies do not have these same views.

— In some cultures, children are viewed as adults as soon as their physical and mental development enables them to perform an adult's job.

— Child sexual exploitation (CSE) produces long-term adverse effects.

— CSE includes both commercial and noncommercial sexual abuse and commonly involves pornography and prostitution.

— The number of US child victims of sexual abuse, assault, and exploitation is estimated to be hundreds of thousands (US Dept of Justice [USDOJ], 2003).

— An estimated quarter million children are sexually exploited for profit in the United States each year.

DEFINITIONS

— *Child pornography*. Photographing children engaged in sexual acts or seductive positions in order to entice the viewer into a sexual response.

— *Child sexual abuse*. Illegal sexual activity involving children younger than 18 years. Usually perpetrated by an adult (Goldstein, 1999).

— *Child sexual assault*. Any sexual act directed against children younger than 8 years, forcibly and/or against their will or when they cannot give consent because of temporary or permanent mental or physical incapacity (Snyder, 2000).

— *Child sexual exploitation*. Practices by which a person (usually an adult) achieves sexual gratification, financial gain, or advancement through abusing or exploiting children's sexuality, abrogating their human right to dignity, equality, autonomy, and physical and mental well-being.

— *Commercial sexual exploitation of children*. Sexual exploitation of children done entirely or primarily for financial or other economic reasons. Second parties benefit from sexual activity with children either by making a profit or through a quid pro quo arrangement.

— *Information and communication technology (ICT)*. All methods of technology presently used in child sexual exploitation, including the Internet, Web cameras, cellular/mobile phones, and iPods.

— *Prostitution*. Engaging in sexual acts for profit.

— *Sex exploiter*. Perpetrator or sex offender; may encompass commercial as well as noncommercial sexual exploitation.

— *Sex tourism*. Visiting other countries for the specific purpose of having sexual relationships with children.

— *Thrownaway children*. Children who have been abandoned or evicted from their family homes.

— *Trafficking*. Transporting individuals for the purpose of sexual exploitation.

VICTIMS

— The Convention on Rights of the Child defines ***childhood*** as continuing up to age 18 years, even if individuals must care for families before the age of 18 years or are married at 10 years of age or younger.

— Factors pertinent to victims that contribute to victimization:

1. *Childhood.* Vulnerability, dependence, lack of power, and the fact that children make fewer emotional demands than adults.

2. *Family situations.* Dysfunction, history of physical or sexual abuse or assault, history of mental illness or substance abuse, poverty, immature decision-making abilities, facilitation of sexual exploitation activities, and criminal or deviant behavior.

3. *Psychosocial factors.* See **Table 1-1**.

4. *Environmental factors.* Demand for children, economic gain, disabilities, violence, child labor, gangs, and devaluing of children.

5. *Other social forces and processes.* See **Table 1-2**.

Table 1-1. Psychosocial Factors Contributing to the Prostitution of Children

— Poverty

— Power and powerlessness

— Lack of knowledge

— Child as a commodity

— Consumerism

— Macho or machismo culture

— Children sexually abused or exploited in the private sphere

— Taboos

— Lack of knowledge regarding the needs of children

— Dysfunctional families

Table 1-2. Factors Contributing to the Commercial Sexual Exploitation of Children and Youths

DOMAIN	DEFINITION	CONTRIBUTING FACTORS
Macro/Contextual (External)	External forces and processes that exist in the larger social environment over which individuals can exercise only minimal control but which, nonetheless, exert a powerful influence on the lives of children and their families.	— Socioeconomic — Societal attitudes toward children and youth — Social anomie among children and youths (ie, a lack of connectedness on the part of youth with the larger society and their place within it) — Poverty — Child victims of crime and violence — Societal responses to crimes committed against children, including sexual crimes — Presence of preexisting adult prostitution "markets" — Presence of groups advocating child-adult sexual relationships — Sexual behavior of unattached and transient males (ie, military personnel, seasonal workers, truckers, motorcycle gangs, conventioneers) — Community knowledge and attitudes concerning HIV/AIDS and other sexually transmitted diseases

Micro/Situational (External)

External forces and processes that **impact children and their families** directly but over which they can exert some measure of control.

— Sociobehavioral
  — **Family dysfunction**
    — Parental drug dependency
    — History of physical and/or sexual assault
    — Personal drug dependency
    — School/other social performance failures
    — Gang membership
  — Active recruitment into prostitution by others
    — Peers
    — Parents or other family members (including siblings)
    — Local pimps
    — National and/or international crime organizations

Individual (Internal)

Psychogenic and cognitive forces that influence a child's sense of mastery over her/his own personal environment and future.

— Psychogenic
  — Poor self-esteem
  — Chronic depression
  — External locus of control
— Seriously restricted future orientation

OFFENDERS

— Offenders can include family members or strangers.

— They are mostly men older than 30 years (see Chapter 2, Victims and Offenders).

— Many are not pedophiles or sadistic, psychopathic criminals.

— They use pornography to desensitize victims to the explicit nature of otherwise unacceptable behavior, stimulate their victims sexually, and lure victims into a secret relationship, sometimes with romantic overtones.

— Seduction can produce loyalty to the offender that the child considers more important than maintaining the family's moral value structure.

— The exploitation process can be accomplished in person or in chat rooms accessed over the Internet in the child's home.

— Pornography often involves family facilitation.

1. Children are rarely sexually abused in pornography production by strangers except in child sex tourism.

2. Pictures and videos may be made by a family member of the victim, then sold or traded to others via the Internet, including commercial Webmasters who post graphics on Web sites that consumers visit for a fee.

— Adults involved in the sex trade continuum of child sexual abuse, the production of child pornography, and child prostitution often employ coercive tactics.

— Adolescent girls who are involved with gangs can be coerced into prostitution to support the gang economy.

FORMS OF CHILD SEXUAL EXPLOITATION

— Exploitation can take place in private, in institutions, or in commercially exploitative contexts (child prostitution, trafficking, or sale of children or child pornography).

— **Table 1-3** lists acts considered sexual abuse by the Economic and Social Commission for Asia and the Pacific (ESCAP, 2000).

— CSE is particularly widespread in Southeast Asia, southern Asia, Latin America, and countries that are developing or that have "transition economies" (Bales, 1999; Caldwell et al, 1997; Estes, 1995, 1996a, 1996b, 1998a; Hughes, 2000; Richard, 1999; Rigi, 2003).

— Child sex tourism occurs in both rich and poor countries.

PORNOGRAPHY

— Pornography is widespread on the Internet, particularly in chat rooms.

— It is available in various media forms (eg, single computer images, video clips, full-length videotapes, audio clips).

Table 1-3. Acts Considered Sexual Abuse

Physical sexual abuse. Touching and fondling of the sexual parts of the child's body (genitals and anus) or touching the breasts of pubescent girls, or the child's touching the sexual parts of a partner's body; sexual kissing and embraces; penetration, which includes penile, digital, and object penetration of the vagina, mouth, or anus; masturbating a child or forcing the child to masturbate the perpetrator

Verbal sexual abuse. Sexual language that is inappropriate for the age of the child used by the perpetrator to generate sexual excitement, including making lewd comments about the child's body and making obscene phone calls

Emotional sexual abuse. Use of a child by a parent or adult to fill inappropriate emotional needs, thereby forcing the child to fulfill the role of a spouse

Exhibitionism and voyeurism. Having a child pose, undress, or perform in a sexual fashion on film or in person (exhibitionism); peeping into bathrooms or bedrooms to spy on a child (voyeurism); exposing children to adult sexual activity or pornographic movies and photographs

Adapted from ESCAP, 2000.

— Child pornography includes commercially made images and videotapes of children from indigent countries.

— A series of child pornography can depict severe child abuse occurring over prolonged periods of time, sometimes in families.

— Victims are often runaways who resort to sexual acts for survival.

— Victims are poorly paid for their services and used only as long as they portray the desired sexual behaviors.

PROSTITUTION
— Prostitution often occurs as an underground, highly mobile, complex network of organized crime.

— It includes escort services.

— It is often not publicly perceived.

— Child and teenaged victims do not choose the life, lacking the knowledge, maturity, and awareness to fully understand their actions and make responsible choices (Minnesota Attorney General's Office, 2000).

OTHER
— Trafficking of women and children for sexual purposes

— Sex tourism, with travel often to Third World countries for the express purpose of having sex with children

— Early marriages, with girls married before puberty

— Temple prostitutes (Devadasi)

— Sugar daddies (phenomenon wherein elderly men provide pocket money for teenaged girls who provide sexual services)

FACTORS INFLUENCING CHILD SEXUAL EXPLOITATION
— Poverty is a key force pushing children onto the streets.

1. Welfare reform can diminish mothers' benefits below what is needed to maintain a home, putting more women and children at risk for homelessness.

2. Boys and young men comprise the majority of homeless individuals.

— A commercial demand exists for children used for sexual purposes.

— Children are devalued by society.

CONSEQUENCES OF CHILD SEXUAL EXPLOITATION

FOR THE CHILD/ADOLESCENT

— Overall poor health

— Skin diseases from being locked up in dark rooms with insufficient oxygen and lack of proper sanitation

— Physical consequences of early pregnancy

— Susceptibility to STDs

— Drug and substance abuse problems

— Psychological problems, including affective disorders, posttraumatic stress disorder, depression, borderline personality disorder, suicidality, and dissociative identity disorder (Farley & Barkan, 1998; Ross et al, 1990)

FOR SOCIETY

— Violence, rape, and homelessness that accompany the life of a prostituted adult

— Stronger federal laws in the United States (**Table 1-4**)

— Policing of the Internet

— Economic impact, especially with Internet pornography, prostitution, trafficking, and sex tourism

---

Table 1-4. Federal Child Pornography Legislation

1977	Protection of Children Against Sexual Exploitation Act
1984	Child Protection Act
1986	Child Sexual Abuse and Pornography Act

(continued)

Table 1-4. *(continued)*

1986	Child Abuse Victims' Rights Act
1988	Child Protection and Obscenity Enforcement Act
1996	Communications Decency Act
1996	Child Pornography Prevention Act
1998	Child Online Protection Act
1998	Protection of Children from Sexual Predators Act
2000	Children's Internet Protection Act
2003	Prosecutorial Remedies and Other Tools to end the Exploitation of Children Today Act (PROTECT Act)

REFERENCES

Bales K. *Disposable People: New Slavery in the Global Economy.* Berkeley, Calif: University of California Press; 1999.

Blankenhorn D. *Fatherless America.* New York, NY: Basic Books; 1995.

Brownback hosts forum on the impact of explicit entertainment on children [press release]. Washington, DC: Sam Brownback, senator from Kansas; July 26, 2001.

Burton DF, Bwanausi C, Johnson J, Moore L. The relationship between traumatic exposure, family dysfunction, and post-traumatic stress symptoms in male juvenile offenders. *J Trauma Stress.* 1994;7: 83-93.

Caldwell G, Galster S, Steinsor N. *Crime & Servitude: An Exposé of the Traffic in Women for Prostitution From the Newly Independent States.* Moscow, Russia: Global Survival Network; 1997.

Committee on Public Education, American Academy of Pediatrics. Sexuality, contraception, and the media. *Pediatrics.* 2001;107(1): 191-194.

Cooley-Quille M, Turner S, Beidel D. The emotional impact of children's exposure to community violence: a preliminary study. *J Am Acad Child Adolesc Psychiatry*. 1995;34:1362-1368.

Dawson JM, Langan PA. *Murder in Families*. Washington, DC: Bureau of Justice Statistics; 1994.

Economic and Social Commission for Asia and the Pacific. *Sexually Abused and Sexually Exploited Children and Youth in the Greater Mekong Sub-Region: A Qualitative Assessment of Their Health Needs and Available Services*. New York, NY: United Nations; 2000.

Estes RJ. Social development trends in Africa: the need for a new development paradigm. *Soc Dev Issues*. 1995;17:18-47.

Estes RJ. Social development trends in Asia, 1970-1994: the challenges of a new century. *Soc Indic Res*. 1996a;37:119-148.

Estes RJ. Social development trends in Latin America, 1970-1994: in the shadows of the 21st century. *Soc Dev Issues*. 1996b;18:25-52.

Estes RJ. Social development trends in the successor states to the former Soviet Union: the search for a new paradigm. In: Kempe RH, ed. *Challenges of Transformation and Transition From Centrally Planned to Market Economies*. UNCRD Research Report Series No. 26. Nagoya, Japan: United Nations Centre for Regional Development. 1998a:13-30.

Farley M, Barkan H. Prostitution, violence, and posttraumatic stress disorder. *Women Health*. 1998;27:37-49.

Gilligan J. *Violence: Our Deadly Epidemic and Its Causes*. New York, NY: Putnam; 1996.

Goldstein SL. *The Sexual Exploitation of Children: A Practical Guide to Assessment, Investigation, and Intervention*. 2nd ed. Boca Raton, Fla: CRC Press; 1999.

Horn WF. *Father Facts*. 3rd ed. Gaithersburg, Md: National Fatherhood Initiative; 1998.

Hughes DM. The "Natasha" trade: the transnational shadow market of trafficking in women. *J Int Aff*. 2000;53:625-652.

Margolin L, Child abuse by mothers' boyfriends: why the overrepresentation? *Child Abuse Negl.* 1992;16(4):541-551.

Minnesota Attorney General's Office. The Hofstede Committee Report: Juvenile Prostitution in Minnesota. 2000. Available at: http://www.ag.state.mn.us/consumer/PDF/hofstede.pdf. Accessed September 29, 2004.

Richard AO. *International Trafficking in Women to the US: A Contemporary Manifestation of Slavery and Organized Crime.* Washington, DC: US State Dept Bureau of Intelligence and Research; 1999.

Rigi J. The conditions of post-Soviet dispossessed youth and work in Almaty, Kazakhstan. *Crit Anthropol.* 2003;23:35-49.

Ross CA, Anderson G, Heber S, Norton GR. Dissociation and abuse among multiple-personality patients, prostitutes, and exotic dancers. *Hosp Community Psychiatry.* 1990;41:328-330.

Sedlak AJ, Broadhurst DD. *The Third National Incidence Study of Child Abuse and Neglect: Final Report.* Washington, DC: US Dept of Health & Human Services; 1996.

Smith C, Thornberry TP. The relationship between childhood maltreatment and adolescent involvement in delinquency. *Criminology.* 1995;33:451-479.

Snyder HN. *Sexual Assault of Young Children as Reported to Law Enforcement: Victim, Incident, and Offender Characteristics—A Statistical Report Using Data from the National Incident-Based Reporting System.* Washington, DC: US Dept of Justice, Office of Justice Programs; 2000.

Sobsey D, Randall W, Parrila RK. Gender differences in abused children with and without disabilities. *Child Abuse Negl.* 1997; 21(8):707-720.

US Department of Health & Human Services. *Survey on Child Health.* Washington, DC: US Dept of Health & Human Services, National Center for Health Statistics; 1993.

US Department of Justice. *Juvenile Offenders and Victims: 2002 National Report.* Washington, DC: US Dept of Justice, Office of Juvenile Justice and Delinquency Prevention; 2003.

Chapter 2

Victims and Offenders

Det Sgt Joseph S. Bova Conti, BA
Lt William D. Carson, MA, SPSC
Peter I. Collins, MCA, MD, FRCP(C)
Richard J. Estes, DSW, ACSW
James A. H. Farrow, MD, FSAM
Mary Anne Layden, PhD
Ethel Quayle, BA, MSc, PsychD
Linnea W. Smith, MD
Max Taylor, PhD, C. Forensic Psychology
Neil Alan Weiner, PhD

— Children may be recruited anywhere there is inadequate adult supervision (eg, malls, entertainment arcades, carnivals, tourist attractions, concerts, and clubs).

— Offenders groom and then seduce the child or adolescent with promises of wealth, luxury, designer clothing, expensive vehicles, or an exciting life.

Victims

— Children are perfect victims: innocent, trusting, and easy prey for predators.

— Vulnerability, lack of parental supervision and family involvement, and societal influences increase susceptibility.

— Child sexual exploitation (CSE) victims are often silent or respond with feigned confidence when confronted.

— Most CSE victims are forced into prostitution, drugs, or pornography (**Table 2-1**).

Table 2-1. Underage Victim Terms: Lolita and Chickenhawk

Lolita, in the parlance of child sexual exploitation, denotes a female who is, or appears to be, a minor. It functions as a code word alerting consumers of child pornography with underage females without otherwise drawing the attention of the public with explicit or graphic terms. This term was derived from the book of the same name by Vladimir Nabokov in which the adult character is sexually attracted to a 13-year-old girl named Lolita.

Chickenhawk is a slang term for underage male victims of sexual exploitation.

TARGETED CHARACTERISTICS OF CHILDREN/ADOLESCENTS

— Alone, troubled, desperate, and unsupervised

— Prepubescent (Note that prepubescence varies because children develop and reach puberty at different ages.)

— Not in school but still want the money and material items of the peer group

— Have older sister or other relative involved in prostitution

— Have various associated factors, including intrafamilial prostitution and/or pornography production

— Live with relative or friend because parents are seperated, divorced, or dead

— Parents are drug addicts, alcoholics, or compulsive gamblers

— Live in extreme poverty, with parents relying on them for income

— Victims of sexual, physical, or emotional abuse

— Homeless, runaways, street youths (**Table 2-2**)

— Lacking the inner strength and aggressiveness to survive on the streets

— Vulnerable to manipulation

— Counterculture youths or those with a bad attitude (rebellious or sarcastic), though this can be unattractive to offenders

— Delinquent and institutional youths

— Unemployed or not receiving regular educational or health services (Gerber, 1997; Klein et al, 2000)

— Lonely, needy, vulnerable, seeking attention, or looking for a friend

— Passive, quiet, naïve, loving, weak, innocent, poor, or neglected

— Low self-esteem

Table 2-2. Typology of Homeless Youths Involved in Survival Sex		
TYPE	DESCRIPTION	RISK FOR SEXUAL EXPLOITATION
Situational runaways	— Short periods away from home — Minor disputes with parents — Runaway behavior often repeated	Low-moderate
Runaways	— Longer periods away from home — Major disputes with parents — Histories of abuse and neglect — Delinquency history	Moderate-high
Thrownaways	— Younger age — Parental neglect and rejection high — In and out of youth shelters	Very high
Systems youths	— Histories of childhood group foster care and institutionalization — History of mental illness and conduct disorders — Vulnerable to dysfunctional living situations on the streets	Very high

PROTECTIVE TRAITS

— Unattractive physical characteristics such as obesity

— Actively involved parents

— Good communication between children and parents

— Aura of confidence, good self-esteem, outgoing personality, and lack of interest in sex talk

— Bad attitude (Some offenders do consider these children easy targets.)

EFFECTS OF CHILDHOOD SEXUAL ABUSE

— Children suffer more negative effects of sexual abuse than adults (Burnam et al, 1988).

— Rates of depression, posttraumatic stress disorder (PTSD), alcohol and drug dependency, phobia, suicidal behavior, anxiety, general impairment in psychological adjustment, borderline personality disorder, generalized anxiety disorder, panic disorder, and eating disorders are higher among victims (Bryer et al, 1987; Burnam et al, 1988; Cheasty et al, 1998; Felitti, 1991; Fergusson et al, 1996; Gorcey et al, 1986; Kendler et al, 2000; MacMillan et al, 2001; McCauley et al, 1997; Mullen et al, 1993; Neumann et al, 1996; Pribor & Dinwiddie, 1992; Stein et al, 1988; Vize & Cooper, 1995; Weiss et al, 1999).

— Adverse outcomes are more likely with more severe or frequent abuse (Briere & Runtz, 1988; Cheasty et al, 1998; Mullen et al, 1993; Walker et al, 1992).

— Negative social consequences include higher rates of teenaged marriage, divorce, separation, and lower socioeconomic status (Bagley & Ramsey, 1985; Bifulco et al, 1991; Mullen et al, 1988).

EFFECTS OF PROSTITUTION

— Extremely high probability of assault (Saikaew, 2001)

— Delinquency

— Drug use and alcoholism

— Promiscuity

— Truancy and running away from home

CONSEQUENCES OF PORNOGRAPHY (KELLY ET AL, 1995)

— Traumatic sexualization

— Betrayal

— Powerlessness

— Reluctance to disclose abuse

— Shame/humiliation (eg, from fear that people will believe they were complicit in the abuse or photography because of their smiling faces)

— Long-term effects of being photographed:

1. Are more debilitating than short-term or mid-term effects.

2. Are compounded when children are involved in more forms of exploitation.

3. Can, for children who are exploited by having their images placed on the Internet, include being tormented by the fact that the images cannot be destroyed and may continue to be used by thousands of people.

4. May be influenced by a child's age at the time the images are produced.

EFFECTS OF TRAUMA ON ADULT SURVIVORS OF CHILD SEXUAL EXPLOITATION

— Trauma beliefs:

1. Trauma beliefs are children's perceptions and interpretations of the trauma and may relate to themselves or others.

2. Children see trauma in terms of their own lovability and power.

3. Issues of trust of others are adversely affected (**Table 2-3**).

— Coping behaviors:

1. Children have fewer coping resources than adults.

2. Children cannot make adults stop doing what they are doing.

3. Beliefs about self and others affect coping behaviors. If children feel bad and worthless, they may deal with it or try to hide the information from others by becoming people pleasers or avoiding people whenever possible (**Table 2-4**).

Table 2-3. Beliefs of Childhood Sexual Industry Victims

BELIEFS ABOUT THEMSELVES: LOVABILITY

— I'm dirty, disgusting, bad, and morally corrupt.
— I'm to blame for what happened to me. I caused it.
— I must have liked what happened to me. If I liked any part of it, it means I liked all of it.
— Sex is the only thing about me that is valuable. Sex is the only currency.
— In order to get others to pay attention to me, I have to use sex. I'm so broken I can't trust my feelings. Others say I like things that I don't think I like.
— If I can get people to have sex with me or to want to have sex with me, it means I am lovable and worthwhile. Sex is lovability.

BELIEFS ABOUT THEMSELVES: POWER

— I'm weak and vulnerable.
— There is nothing I can do to make my situation better.
— I have no right or am unable to tell others that I don't want to have sex with them, and they wouldn't stop even if I did. I can't protect my boundaries or stop or limit the visual or physical invasion.
— If I get people to have sex with me or to want to have sex with me, it means I am powerful. Sex is power.

BELIEFS ABOUT OTHERS: TRUST

— Other people will use me, abuse me, take advantage of me, and then leave me.
— People you think you can trust or who are the most intimate with you hurt you the most.
— Other people will find out what happened to me and judge me or hurt me because of it.
— Don't expect sex, love, and long-term commitment to be connected. People will never love me, and they will always leave. Take sex as a substitute.
— Others only want sex from me and they want to hurt me. Sex and violence are connected.

Table 2-4. Coping Strategies of Childhood Sexual Exploitation Industry Victims

— Pleasing others	— Clinging	— Denial
— Harming self	— Self-medicating with drugs and/or alcohol	— Dissociating
— Dependency		— Sex
— Enmeshment	— Avoidance	— Aggression
— Underfunctioning	— Distancing	
— Passivity	— Overfunctioning	

— Missing life skills:

1. Abused children do not learn certain skills while growing up and lack other life choices.

2. Children should learn life skills to help them successfully negotiate the adult world (**Table 2-5**).

3. These skills are learned by watching parents. For victims of the CSE industry this is often impossible.

— Psychiatric outcomes: **Table 2-6**.

Table 2-5. Missing Life Skills of Childhood Sexual Exploitation Industry Victims

— Intimacy	— Decision-making
— Trust-judgment	— Communication
— Boundary protection	— Self-soothing
— Parenting	— Affect modulation
— Problem-solving	— Employment

Table 2-6. Adult Psychological Disorders of Childhood Sexual Exploitation Industry Victims

— Depression
— Generalized anxiety disorder
— Panic disorder
— Posttraumatic stress disorder
— Eating disorders

— Substance abuse disorders
— Avoidant personality disorder
— Dependent personality disorder
— Borderline personality disorder

CHILDHOOD SEXUAL ABUSE AND LATER PROSTITUTION
— 28% to 65% of prostituted teenagers were sexually abused (Seng, 1989).

— 57% of prostituted adults were sexually assaulted as children (Farley & Barkan, 1998).

— Prostituted adults are more likely to have been victims of incest, to have experienced physical force during their first intercourse, to be raped, and to experience multiple rapes (James & Meyerding, 1977).

— Prostituted adults report lives marked by violence (82%), rape (68%), and homelessness (84%).

— Prostitution reduces the likelihood of ever marrying.

— Prostituted adults have higher rates of psychological problems: PTSD, depression, substance abuse, borderline personality disorder, suicidality, and dissociative identity disorder (Farley & Barkan, 1998; Ross et al, 1990).

— 88% of Prostituted adults want to leave their life of prostitution.

OFFENDERS
— The persons who exploit children sexually are most often men, but some child sex crimes are committed by women, couples, and other juveniles (De Albuquerque, 1999; National Center on Child Abuse and Neglect, 2003; Righthand & Welch, 2001; Simmons, 1996;

Snyder, 2000; US Dept of Health & Human Services [USDHHS], 2003; US Dept of Justice, 2003).

— Sexual predators can be young, old, well-educated, poorly educated, and as likely to come from middle America as from coastal cities.

— Except for child pornography, organized criminal enterprises usually avoid involvement in the commercial sexual exploitation of children aged 10 years or younger because such young children are difficult to control and carry high risks.

PARAPHILIAS

— *Paraphilias* are abnormal, unusual, or deviant sexual preferences directed toward a particular target or abnormal activity (Freund et al, 1997).

— The diagnostic criteria for paraphilias (*Diagnostic and Statistical Manual of Mental Disorders* [DSM-IV-TR]) include:

1. Experiencing recurrent and intense sexually arousing fantasies, urges, or behavior directed toward body parts or nonhuman objects; suffering or humiliation of either partner during the sex act; or taking part in sexual activity with a nonconsenting person.

2. Experiencing clinically significant distress or impairment of functioning as a result of fantasies, urges, or behaviors (American Psychiatric Association, 2000).

— **Tables 2-7** and **2-8** list various paraphilias.

— Most individuals with a paraphilia do not seek help.

— Individuals usually become aware of deviant sexual interests around puberty but may not act on fantasies for years, if at all.

— Treatment is usually postarrest and on a judicial order or at the request of a sexual partner who cannot tolerate the unconventional sexual activities.

— Average time between onset of the paraphilia and receiving treatment is 12 years.

Table 2-7. Common Paraphilias

PARAPHILIA	PREFERRED ACTIVITY OR TARGET
Exhibitionism	Exposing one's genitals to an unsuspecting woman or child
Fetishism	Erotic attraction to a nonliving object
Frotteurism	Rubbing up against a nonconsenting person
Pedophilia	Prepubescent children
Masochism	Being humiliated, bound, or made to suffer
Sadism	Psychological or physical suffering of the target
Transvestic fetishism	Cross-dressing
Voyeurism	Observing unsuspecting individuals who are disrobing, naked, or engaging in sexual activity

Table 2-8. Examples of Clinically Identified Paraphilias

PARAPHILIA	STIMULUS
Acrotomophilia	Stump of an amputee and/or the desire to amputate someone's limb
Apotemnophilia	Self-amputation (or done in a hospital)
Asphyxiophilia	Self-induced asphyxiation almost to the point of unconsciousness; also known as auto-erotic asphyxiation
Autoassassinophilia	Managing the possibility of one's own masochistic death
Autonepiophilia	Impersonating a baby in diapers
Biastophilia	Rape preference
Coprophilia	Handling, being smeared with, or ingesting feces
Klismaphilia	Receiving or giving enemas
Morphophilia	A particular body type or size

(continued)

Table 2-8. *(continued)*

PARAPHILIA	STIMULUS
Mysophilia	Smelling, chewing, or otherwise using soiled (urine, fecal material, menstrual discharge) or sweaty clothing
Necrophilia	A corpse, or someone acting as though they were dead
Partialism	Particular body part (eg, feet, neck, abdomen)
Scotophilia	Watching others engage in masturbation or sexual intercourse
Stigmatophilia	A partner who has been tattooed, scarified, or pierced in the genital area
Triolism	Observing one's partner engaging in sex with another person
Urophilia	Being urinated on and/or drinking urine
Zoophilia	Engaging in sex with animals

— Most criminal paraphilics have committed 44 crimes a year before their arrest (Abel et al, 1985).

— Some paraphilias (voyeurism, exhibitionism, frotteurism, and rape preference) are theorized as disorders of courtship.

— Often co-occur and are termed *cross-over sexual offenses* because victims are from multiple age, gender, and relationship categories (Heil et al, 2003).

— The Internet provides paraphilics with a high-tech way of pursuing their activities.

PEDOPHILIA

General Information

Technically, pedophilia is a psychiatric diagnosis and can be found in the DSM-IV-TR (see **Table 2-9**) (American Psychiatric Association, 2000).

Table 2-9. Criteria for the Diagnosis of Pedophilia

A. Over a period of at least 6 months, a person has experienced recurrent, intense, sexually arousing fantasies, sexual urges, or behaviors involving sexual activity with a prepubescent child or children (generally age 18 years or younger).

B. The person has acted on these urges, or the sexual urges or fantasies caused marked distress or interpersonal difficulty.

C. The person is at least 16 years of age and at least 5 years older than the child or children in criterion A.

Data from the American Psychiatric Association, 2000.

— Pedophilia is a sexual orientation.

1. Individuals who obsess and fantasize about having sex with prepubescent children are *pedophiles* or *preferential child molesters*, regardless of whether they ever act on the fantasies.

2. A person can be a pedophile and never molest a child.

— *Child molester* describes any person who has ever molested a child, regardless of whether the person is attracted to children.

1. A person can be a child molester and not a pedophile.

2. Some child molesters are situational offenders; they do not prefer children but will molest a child under certain circumstances.

— Pedophiles attracted exclusively to boys (male-target pedophiles) differ from pedophiles attracted only to girls (female-target pedophiles).

— Pedophiles tend to lead a secretive lifestyle.

1. Some are married, have a family, and have a successful business or career and fear the consequences of acting out their desires.

2. Some pedophiles suppress their sexual urges.

3. Some pedophiles seek out partners who look young but are of legal age.

4. Others live a life of fantasy and masturbation, collect child erotica or pornography, and work with or associate with children in a nonsexual way but never have sexual contact with children.

5. Some pedophiles act out sexually with children but never get caught or exposed.

6. Some pedophiles are not reported to law enforcement officials. The issues are handled informally within families, neighborhoods, and organizations.

7. Other pedophiles are reported to the police but not prosecuted for various reasons.

8. Some pedophiles are exposed, arrested, and prosecuted.

9. A convicted pedophile might not serve time in prison, receiving probation or "shock time" (a short sentence, usually 90 to 120 days, to let the offender experience incarceration) instead.

— Many child molesters were molested as children. However, most sexually abused children do not grow up to become pedophiles.

— The cause of pedophilia is complicated and involves an integration of multiple factors (Finkelhor & Araji, 1986).

Common Characteristics of Pedophiles (Lowenstein, 2001; Prentky et al, 1997)

— Personal characteristics:

1. Deficits in social competence (inadequate social and interpersonal skills, lack of assertiveness, low self-esteem)

2. Lack of impulse control

3. Obsessive-compulsive tendencies

4. Lack of empathy toward children

5. Depression

6. Poor family relations

7. First experience as a perpetrator is likely at a younger age (**Figure 2-1**)

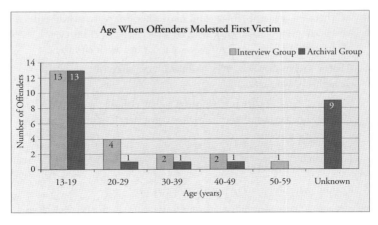

Figure 2-1. *Comparison of offenders in interview and archival groups as related to when they molested their first victim.*

— Pedophilia is not linked to education, employment, or volunteer affiliations.

— 2 age variant preferences:

1. *Infantaphilia* is erotic attraction to children aged 5 years or younger.

2. *Hebephilia* or *ephebophilia* is sexual attraction to children who have reached puberty and are in the early stages of adolescence.

3. In both, the immature body parts are sexually arousing.

— *Exclusive pedophiles* are men who can have sex only with children.

— *Nonexclusive pedophiles* are men capable of having age-appropriate sexual relations but who fantasize about sexual contact with children.

— Some pedophiles target single mothers, entering a relationship in order to abuse the children. They may meet in Internet chat rooms as well as dating and singles sites.

— Some pedophiles are attracted equally to boys and girls but most prefer one gender.

OTHER PARAPHILIAS
Zoophilia (Bestiality)
— ***Zoophilia*** involves using animals as sexual objects, including fellatio, cunnilingus, coitus, and masturbation.

— It can occur opportunistically or as a preferred sexual practice.

— Treated individuals are usually under the influence of alcohol or drugs, psychopaths, or cognitively impaired. A few are psychotics (Bluglass, 1990).

— ***Formicophilia*** focuses on small creatures that creep, crawl, or nibble on the body, especially sexually significant sites.

Fetishism
— A ***fetish*** is an inanimate object or part of the body (partialism) with great erotic meaning for the person (Binet, 1887).

— A ***souvenir*** is an item taken from a victim as a reminder of a pleasurable encounter; it may be used for masturbatory fantasies.

— Use of a fetish item may become requisite for any sexual activity.

— Sometimes it is the texture of the material that arouses.

— The most common fetishes are female undergarments or lingerie. Worn garments soiled with urine or feces are particularly desirable.

— Web sites or chat rooms devoted to various fetishes are available where "fetters" can communicate with individuals having similar deviant interests.

— The Diaper Pail Fraternity is composed of individuals erotically aroused by wearing diapers and acting like babies.

1. Members prefer to call themselves "adult babies" or "diaperists."

2. They order adult-size diapers, pacifiers, and other items in order to act out their erotic fantasies.

3. The behavior can consist of being disciplined, spanked, or restrained and often is associated with urophilia or coprophilia.

— Individuals may break into residences or steal the garbage from houses where they know a baby is in the residence and then use soiled diapers as masturbatory aids.

Urophilia, Coprophilia, and Klismaphilia

— These paraphilias are linked to pedophilia acting out.

— Activities involve being urinated upon (golden showers), observing others urinating, drinking urine, drinking urine out of toilets where children have voided, or collecting the urine of victims.

— These paraphilias can be associated with sadomasochistic behavior (Denson, 1982) or with demeaning the victim after a sexual attack.

— Offenders engaged in coprophilia have a sexual fascination with the use of feces in sexual activities, including smelling, eating, or smearing feces on the body.

— Practitioners of klismaphilia are erotically aroused by giving or receiving enemas.

Sadism and Hyperdominance

— The sadist obtains sexual pleasure by inflicting pain and suffering.

— Features of sexual sadism include cruelty, torture, sexual mutilation of the victim, and sexual interest in sadistic acts (Marshall & Yates, 2004).

— Hyperdominant sexual activity (bondage) is often found in child pornography images on the Internet.

— The combination of sadism and pedophilia can be lethal.

— Sadism is more prevalent in nonfamilial contact offenses.

— Sexual homicides of children are rare but are often the work of a sadist.

— Nonsadistic pedophiles may kill a child out of fear of being caught. If the body is subsequently dismembered by the nonsadistic pedophile, it is regarded as defensive dismemberment (Rajs et al, 1998).

— A *snuff film* is a homemade movie or video allegedly depicting an actual murder for entertainment purposes.

Picquerism

— Involves erotic arousal generated by poking with a sharp object or ritualistic stabbing of the victim for sexual pleasure.

— Practitioners may draw images of arrows, spears, or knives on pictures of children or make videotapes of nude children having hypodermic needles inserted in their buttocks.

Necrophilia

— 2 types (Rosman & Resnick, 1988):

1. *Necrophilia*. Sexual attraction to corpses.

2. *Pseudonecrophilia*. Corpses act as a sexual substitute.

— Behavior of necrophiliacs:

1. Can involve kissing, fondling, or performing cunnilingus on the body as well as intercourse (Hucker, 1990)

2. May steal pubic hair

3. May mutilate the body and engage in necrophagia (eating of corpses or body parts of corpses)

— Necrophilia is rare, but with no victims to complain, it is likely underreported.

RECRUITMENT PROCESS

— Tools include isolation, coercion, threats, minimization of the act, grooming, emotional abuse, intimidation, social status, and overt violence.

— Key components in exploitation are power and control.

— Techniques:

1. Entice, groom, and gain the confidence of the child.

2. Psychologically and physically gain power and control over the child to force the child into prostitution.

3. Move the child from state to state and force the child to work as a prostitute in areas where police and social workers have less experience with the prostitution of children.

GROOMING

See **Table 2-10**.

— Grooming lasts for variable lengths of time before sexual abuse occurs.

— Grooming can involve borderline, or "accidental," touching to assess the child's reaction.

1. Gradual process moves from normal physical touching to overt sexual acts.

2. Subtle changes can occur without the child realizing what is happening.

— Grooming includes rationalizations and assurances that sexual activities are natural and acceptable.

1. Male pedophiles who molest boys minimize the homosexual aspect, making activities seem like experimentation and play. They reassure boys that performing these acts does not mean the boys or offenders are homosexuals.

2. Boys may not report sexual abuse because of embarrassment and the stigma associated with homosexual activities, and they may feel guilt and shame because they were aroused by the contact or think of themselves as willing participants.

3. Pedophiles can give boys off-limit items (cigarettes, alcohol, drugs, pornography) to entrap them further.

Table 2-10. Steps in Grooming a Victim

Step 1: Offender cultivates a trusting relationship with the child.

Step 2: Offender provides special attention, affection, favors, money, and gifts.

Step 3: Offender and victim share intimate or personal secrets or have sexual conversations disguised as educational.

Step 4: Predator assesses child's vulnerabilities and weaknesses, taking advantage of natural curiosity about sex, and then lowers inhibitions.

— The grooming and seduction process creates a strong bond and loyalty between victim and offender. Some molested children do not consider themselves victims.

— Most offenders carefully observe body language and gauge reactions to touch and conversation to determine if it is safe to proceed.

— Once it is determined that the boy is not interested, most offenders discontinue their approaches.

Types of Exploitation

In the Home

— Sex crimes committed against children in their own homes rarely involve a commercial aspect.

— These instances tend to be opportunistic and involve offenders known to the child, the family, or both (USDHHS, 2003).

— Web cameras can be used to groom children and youths in the home to become compliant victims.

Not in the Home

— Sex crimes committed against street children are nearly always economic or commercial in nature.

— The child exchanges sex for money or something else of commercial value.

— Offenders are rarely known to the child or the child's family and typically perceive the child as a temporary means to satisfy a need.

— Offenders rarely develop long-lasting relationships with their victims; many express affection but only to obtain cooperation.

— Categories of child sexual exploiters not in the home:

1. Pedophiles

2. Transient males, including members of the military, truck drivers, seasonal workers, conventioneers, and sex tourists

3. Opportunistic exploiters (people who sexually abuse whoever is available for sex, including children)

4. Pimps

5. Traffickers

6. Other juveniles

On the Internet (Pornography)
— Individuals identified in trading abusive images are the producer, the trader, and the collector. Categories may overlap.

1. Collectors can be active (directly communicating with other people through Internet relay chat) or passive (accessing images through protocols not requiring direct access to other people, such as Web sites). (See **Figures 3-1** and **3-2** in Chapter 3, Child Pornography.)

2. Individuals move between the different roles as inclination and opportunity allow (Quayle & Taylor, 2003).

3. In general, no money changes hands; a form of barter is used.

4. Access to pay Web sites requires payment to the Web site owner.

— Characteristics of offenders who access Internet abuse images:

1. All ages and all social backgrounds

2. Various degrees of technical sophistication

3. Known sexual offenders and others with no previous acknowledged sexual interest in children

4. No published accounts of women offending on the Internet

— Offenders make objects of the photographs, treating the images as collectibles. They may edit images to remove features of no interest (including the face).

1. Many people who access and distribute child pornography have no history of pursuing sexual contact or relationships with real children (Quayle et al, 2000).

2. The Internet may facilitate interests in children not previously expressed.

Trafficking
— Adult traffickers include amateur traffickers, small groups of organized criminals, and multilayered trafficking networks organized both nationally and internationally (Graycar, 1999; Lederer, 2001; Richard, 1999; Schloenhardt, 1999; US Dept of State [USDOS], 2003; Yoon, 1997).

— Trafficking functionaries: **Table 2-11**.

Category	Roles
Arrangers/investors	Invest money in the operation and oversee the criminal organization. Rarely known to lower-level employees or migrants being trafficked. Not easily connected with specific crimes.
Recruiters	Middlemen between arrangers and customers. Find and mobilize potential migrants and collect money. Those in country of departure do not usually know exact trafficking passage and are not permanent employees. Often come from the same area as the migrants and share their culture.
Transporter providers and operators	Assist migrants leaving country of origin. Those in destination country bring undocumented immigrants from airport, seaport, or coast to large cities. Position requires technical sophistication to change operations in reaction to law enforcement and coastal surveillance activities. They seldom know criminal structure, maintaining contact through intermediaries.
Corrupt public officials (bribable protectors)	Paid to obtain travel documents for customers. Law enforcement persons accept bribes so migrants can enter and exit countries illegally. May also protect the criminal organization through position, status, privileges, etc.

(continued)

Table 2-11. *(continued)*

CATEGORY	ROLES
Informers	Gather information on border surveillance, immigration and transit procedures and regulations, asylum systems, and law enforcement. Use information to facilitate trafficking activities. Sometimes a core group of informers manage information flow and access well-organized and centralized communications systems through sophisticated technology.
Guides and crew members	Move illegal migrants from one transit point to the other or help migrants enter country. Crew members charter trafficking vessels and accompany migrants throughout the passage.
Enforcers	Often also illegal migrants; primarily police the staff and migrants and maintain order, often using violence.
Supporting personnel and specialists	Usually local people in transit points who provide housing and other assistance to illegal migrants. Some are skilled workers who provide specialized products and services. Usually paid for casual duties only. Included are taxi drivers; operators of "safe houses"; persons who prepare false or stolen documents; "coyotes" who cross into the United States with children at border points; persons who provide housing and sometimes jobs as domestics or in restaurants or bars; and those who introduce children to the persons who bought them or own their contract.
Debt collectors	Persons who collect trafficking fees. Based in destination country.
Money movers	Experts at laundering criminal proceeds, disguising their origin through various transactions or investing in legitimate businesses.

REFERENCES

Abel GG, Becker JV, Mittleman M. Sexual offenders: results of assessment and recommendations for treatment. In: Ben-Aron MH, Hucker Sj, Webster CD, eds. *Clinical Criminology: Current Concept.* Toronto, Canada: M & M Graphics; 1985:191-205.

American Psychiatric Association. *Diagnostic and Statistical Manual of Mental Disorders.* 4th ed. Text revision. Washington, DC: American Psychiatric Association; 2000.

Bagley C, Ramsey R. Sexual abuse in childhood: psychosocial outcomes and implications for social work practice. *J Soc Work Hum Sex.* 1985;4:33-48.

Bifulco A, Brown GW, Adler Z. Early sexual abuse and clinical depression in adult life. *Br J Psychiatry.* 1991;159:115-122.

Binet A. Du fétishism dans l'amour. *Revue Philosophique.* 1887; 24:142-167.

Bluglass R. Bestiality. In: Bluglass R, Bowden P, Walker N, eds. *Principles and Practice of Forensic Psychiatry.* London, England: Churchill Livingstone; 1990:671-676.

Briere J, Runtz M. Symptomatology associated with childhood sexual victimization in a nonclinical adult sample. *Child Abuse Negl.* 1988; 12:51-59.

Bryer JB, Nelson BA, Miller JB, Krol PA. Childhood sexual and physical abuse as factors in adult psychiatric illness. *Am J Psychiatry.* 1987;144:1426-1430.

Burnam MA, Stein JA, Golding JM, et al. Sexual assault and mental disorders in a community population. *J Consult Clin Psychol.* 1988; 56:443-450.

Cheasty M, Clare AW, Collins C. Relation between sexual abuse in childhood and adult depression: case-control study. *BMJ.* 1998;6: 198-201.

De Albuquerque K. Sex, beach boys, and female tourists in the Caribbean. In: Dank B, Refinetti R, eds. *Sex Work and Sex Workers:*

Sexuality & Culture. Vol 1. New Brunswick, NJ: Transaction Publishers; 1999.

Denson R. Undinism: the fetishization of urine. *Can J Psychiatry.* 1982;27:336-338.

Farley M, Barkan H. Prostitution, violence, and posttraumatic stress disorder. *Women Health.* 1998;27:37-49.

Felitti VJ. Long-term medical consequences of incest, rape and molestation. *South Med J.* 1991;84:328-331.

Fergusson DM, Horwood LJ, Lynskey MT. Childhood sexual abuse and psychiatric disorder in young adulthood: II. Psychiatric outcomes of childhood sexual abuse. *Am Acad Child Adolesc Psychiatry.* 1996; 35:1365-1374.

Finkelhor D, Araji S. Explanation of pedophilia: a four factor model. *J Sex Res.* 1986;22(2):145-161.

Freund K, Seto M, Kuban M. Frotteurism and the theory of courtship disorder. In: Laws DR, O'Donahue W, eds. *Sexual Deviance: Theory, Assessment and Treatment.* New York, NY: Guilford Press; 1997: 111-113.

Gerber GM. Barriers to health care for street youth. *J Adolesc Health.* 1997;21(5):287-290.

Gorcey M, Santiago JM, McCall-Perez F. Psychological consequences for women sexually abused in childhood. *Soc Psychiatry.* 1986;21: 129-133.

Graycar A. Trafficking in human beings. Paper presented at: International Conference on Migration, Culture, and Crime; July 7, 1999; Israel.

Heil P, Ahlmeyer S, Simons D. Crossover sex offenses. *Sex Abuse.* 2003;15(4):221-236.

Hucker S. Necrophilia and other unusual philias. In: Bluglass R, Bowden P, Walker N, eds. *Principles and Practice of Forensic Psychiatry.* London, England: Churchill Livingstone; 1990:671-676.

James J, Meyerding J. Early sexual experience and prostitution. *Am J Psychiatry*. 1977;134:1381-1385.

Kelly L, Wingfield R, Burton S, Regan L. *Splintered Lives: Sexual Exploitation of Children in the Context of Children's Rights and Child Protection*. London, England: Barnardos; 1995.

Kendler KS, Bulik CM, Silberg J, Hettema JM, Myers J, Prescott CA. Childhood sexual abuse and adult psychiatric and substance use disorders in women: an epidemiological and cotwin control analysis. *Arch Gen Psychiatry*. 2000;57:953-959.

Klein JD, Woods AH, Wilson KM, Prospero M, Greene J, Ringwalt C. Homeless and runaway youths' access to health care. *J Adolesc Health*. 2000;27(5):331-339.

Lederer L. *Human Rights Report on Trafficking of Women and Children*. Baltimore, Md: Johns Hopkins University, The Paul H. Nitze School of Advanced International Studies; 2001.

Lowenstein LF. The identification and diagnosis of alleged victims and alleged pedophiles (what to do and what to avoid doing.) *Police J*. 2001;74(3):237-250.

MacMillan HL, Fleming JE, Streiner DL, et al. Childhood abuse and lifetime psychopathology in a community sample. *Am J Psychiatry*. 2001;158:1878-1883.

Marshall WL, Yates P. Diagnostic issues in sexual sadism among sexual offenders. *J Sex Aggress*. 2004; 10:21-27.

McCauley J, Kern DE, Kolodner K, et al. Clinical characteristic of women with a history of childhood abuse: unhealed wounds. *JAMA*. 1997;277:1362-1368.

Mullen PE, Martin JL, Anderson JC, Romans SE, Herbison GP. Childhood sexual abuse and mental health in adult life. *Br J Psychiatry*. 1993;163:721-732.

Mullen PE, Romans-Clarkson SE, Walton VA, Herbison GP. Impact of sexual and physical abuse on women's mental health. *Lancet*. 1988;1:841-845.

National Center on Child Abuse and Neglect. *Child Maltreatment, 2001*. Washington, DC: Administration for Children and Families of the US Dept of Health and Human Services; 2003.

Neumann DA, Houskamp BM, Pollack VE, Briere J. The long-term sequelae of childhood sexual abuse in women: a meta-analytic review. *Child Maltreat*. 1996;1:6-16.

Prentky RA, Knight RA, Lee AF. *Child Sexual Molestation: Research Issues*. Washington, DC: National Institute of Justice; 1997.

Pribor EF, Dinwiddie SH. Psychiatric correlates of incest in childhood. *Am J Psychiatry*. 1992;149:52-56.

Quayle E, Holland G, Linehan C, Taylor M. The Internet and offending behaviour: a case study. *J Sex Aggress*. 2000;6(1/2):78-96.

Quayle E, Taylor M. Model of problematic Internet use in people with a sexual interest in children. *Cyberpsychol Behav*. 2003;6(1):93-106.

Rajs J, Lundström M, Broberg M, Lidberg L, Lindquest O. Criminal mutilation of the human body in Sweden—a thirty-year medicolegal and forensic study. *J Forensic Sci*. 1998;43:563-580.

Richard AL. *International Trafficking in Women to the US: A Contemporary Manifestation of Slavery and Organized Crime*. Washington, DC: US State Dept Bureau of Intelligence and Research; 1999.

Righthand S, Welch C. *Juveniles Who Have Sexually Offended: A Review of the Professional Literature*. Washington, DC: US Dept of Justice, Office of Juvenile Justice and Delinquency Prevention; 2001.

Rosman J, Resnick P. Necrophilia: an analysis of 122 cases involving paraphilic acts and fantasies. *Bull Am Acad Psychiatry Law*. 1988; 17:153-163.

Ross CA, Anderson G, Heber S, Norton GR. Dissociation and abuse among multiple-personality patients, prostitutes, and exotic dancers. *Hosp Community Psychiatry*. 1990;41:328-330.

Saikaew L. *The Report on Child Prostitution as a Form of Forced Labor: A Non-Governmental Organization Perspective*. Washington, DC: Bureau of International Labor Affairs; 2001.

Schloenhardt A. The business of migration: organized crime and illegal migration in Australia and the Asia-Pacific region. Paper presented at: University of Adelaide Law School; May, 1999; Adelaide, Australia.

Seng MJ. Child sexual abuse and adolescent prostitution: a comparison analysis. *Adolescence.* 1989;24:665-675.

Simmons MJ. Hookers, hustlers, and round-trip vacationers: the gender dynamics of sex and romance Tourism. Paper presented at: Society for the Study of Social Problems; August, 1996; New York, NY.

Snyder HN. *Sexual Assault of Young Children as Reported to Law Enforcement: Victims, Incident, and Offender Characteristics A Statistical Report Using Data from the National Incident-Based Reporting System.* Washington, DC: US Dept of Justice, Office of Justice Programs; 2000.

Stein JA, Golding JM, Siegel JM, Burnam MA, Sorenson SB. Long-term psychological sequelae of child sexual abuse. In: Wyatt GE, Powell GJ, eds. *Lasting Effects of Child Sexual Abuse.* Newbury Park, Calif: Sage Publications; 1988:135-154.

US Department of Health and Human Services. *Perpetrators of child maltreatment, 1997-2001.* Washington, DC: US Dept of Health & Human Services, Administration for Children & Families; 2003. Available at: http://www.acf.hhs.gov/programs/cb/publications/cm01/chapterfour.htm. Accessed March 15, 2004.

US Department of Justice. *Juvenile Offenders and Victims: 2002 National Report.* Washington, DC: US Dept of Justice, Office of Juvenile Justice and Delinquency Prevention; 2003.

US Department of State. *Trafficking in persons report.* Washington, DC: US Dept of State; July, 2003.

Vize CM, Cooper PJ. Sexual abuse in patients with eating disorders, patients with depression and normal controls: a comparative study. *Br J Psychiatry.* 1995;167:80-85.

Walker EA, Katon WJ, Hansom J, et al. Medical and psychiatric symptoms in women with childhood sexual abuse. *Psychosom Med.* 1992;54:658-664.

Weiss EL, Longhurst JG, Mazure CM. Childhood sexual abuse as a risk factor for depression in women: psychological and neurobiological correlates. *Am J Psychiatry*. 1999;156:816-828.

Yoon Y. *International Sexual Slavery*. Washington, DC: CG Issue Overviews; 1997.

Chapter 3

CHILD PORNOGRAPHY

Duncan T. Brown, Esq
Peter I. Collins, MCA, MD, FRCP(C)
Sharon W. Cooper, MD, FAAP
Shyla R. Lefever, PhD
Ethel Quayle, BA, MSc, PsychD
Max Taylor, PhD, C. Forensic Psychology
Bruce Watson, LLB, CA

BACKGROUND

— Child pornography is a photographic record of child sexual abuse. Pornographic images of an actual child cannot be created without sexually exploiting and molesting the child.

— Synthetic pornography involves computer-generated images that may combine a child's face with an adult body or vice versa or may combine several children so images are not of a single identifiable child.

— Pornography's purpose is sexual arousal.

1. Used to lower children's natural resistance to performing sexual acts.

2. Used as an instruction manual to teach children behaviors that are foreign to them.

— Pornography is routinely described as the earliest and most consistent commercial success on the Internet.

1. Child pornography and pedophiliac activity are particularly dangerous to children when the materials and activities are online.

2. The combination of children's natural innocence and sense of security makes them vulnerable to victimization (see Chapter 2, Victims and Offenders).

3. Anonymity provided by the Internet and instant access to people of like deviancies makes exchanging photographs, videos, and audiotapes of child exploitation easy (see Chapter 5, Cyber-Enticement and Internet Travelers).

— Pedophiles collect child pornography (Durkin, 1997; Quayle & Taylor, 2002):

1. To fuel sexual fantasies or serve as a masturbatory aid or prelude to sexual activity. Even nonpornographic or nonsexualized images can be erotically arousing to pedophiles.

2. To validate that the shared sexual preference is common. Most images portray smiling, compliant children, contributing to supposed appropriateness and validation.

DEFINITIONS

— The term *abuse images* is gaining acceptance among professionals.

— *Pornography* is a term with complex connotations, allowing comparison with the depictions of consensual sexual activity between adults. With children there can be no question of consent.

— Combating Paedophile Information Networks in Europe (COPINE) views images as evidentiary material and seeks to develop systematic assessment and intervention approaches.

1. Defines 10 types (levels) of images attractive to adults with a sexual interest in children (**Tables 3-1** and **3-2**)

2. The ascending series of categories broadly reflect degrees of victimization. In most jurisdictions, levels from 5 or 6 upward are illegal.

3. Countries may define illegality differently, especially when unclothed children are involved.

— Some images attractive to an adult with a sexual interest in children may fall outside the legal definition of child pornography. Many images are sexually arousing for a fantasizing individual but may not be explicitly sexual and therefore illegal.

Table 3-1. The COPINE Typology of Abusive Images of Children

LEVEL	DESCRIPTION
1	Indicative (nonerotic/nonsexualized images)
2	Nudist (naked or semi-naked children in legitimate settings)
3	Erotica (surreptitious images showing underwear/nakedness)
4	Posing (deliberate posing suggesting sexual content)
5	Erotic posing (deliberate sexual provocative posing)
6	Explicit erotic posing (emphasis on genital area)
7	Explicit sexual activity not involving adult
8	Assault (involving adult)
9	Gross assault (penetrative assault involving adult)
10	Sadistic/bestiality (sexual images involving pain or animals)

Adapted from Taylor et al, 2001.

Table 3-2. The UK Court of Appeals Sentencing Guidelines Scale Derived From the COPINE Typology

LEVEL	DESCRIPTION
1	COPINE levels 5 and 6
2	COPINE level 7
3	COPINE level 8
4	COPINE level 9
5	COPINE level 10

Adapted from Taylor et al, 2001.

RANGE OF IMAGES

— Range lies along a continuum.

— Range is expressed as a degree or level of victimization.

— Nature of the victimization shown can reflect pedophile's level of engagement with the material and provide visible evidence of sexual fantasy or assault.

— Individuals who participate in trading abuse images are producers, traders, and collectors (see Chapter 2, Victims and Offenders, and **Figure 3-1**) (Quayle & Taylor, 2003).

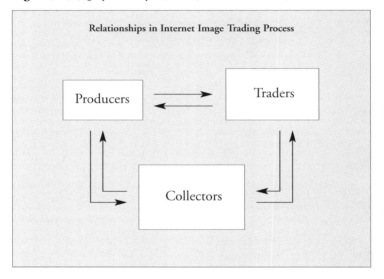

Figure 3-1. *A possible relationship between trading, collecting, and producing abuse images of children.*

SPEECH ISSUES

— 2 types of speech are considered in child pornography.

1. Graphic images or descriptions of children engaged in sexually explicit conduct:

   A. Includes photographs, computer images, magazines, books, or other materials that portray, illustrate, or depict children engaged in sexually explicit conduct.

    B. Are usually stored on a defendant's hard drive or in print media.

    C. Are the object of countless Web sites and chat rooms dedicated to distributing, producing, and amassing child pornography.

2. Communication used by offenders incidental to criminal activities:

    A. Creates conspiracies and aiders and abettors.

    B. Is used by organized and centralized groups to plan strategies for seducing victims (North American Man/Boy Love Association [NAMBLA], 1991) or to build structured networks of pedophiles and molesters to trade or distribute pornography.

    C. Is also used by groups to trade or produce pornography casually in chat rooms or on Web sites.

— Neither type of speech is protected by the First Amendment's guaranty of freedom of speech. Child pornography differs from adult obscenity in that it is clearly defined by statute and is not subject to nebulous or vague tests based on community standards of what is impermissibly obscene.

FORMS AND USES

— Pornographic messages have a strong, negative influence that can affect attitudes and thus also behavior.

1. Messages promote attitudes toward women that support sexual harassment and destroy relationships.

2. The attitudes toward sexuality breed promiscuity and irresponsible sexual behaviors, leading to the spread of sexually transmitted diseases.

3. Images model self-gratification at the expense of others.

4. By showing resistant children photographs of other children engaged in sexual activities, pedophiles convince potential victims that sexual acts are normal activities children will or should enjoy (Densen-Gerber & Hutchinson, 1979).

— Some international organizations, such as NAMBLA, promote organized pornographic freedom.

1. NAMBLA officers and members promote and advocate adult men and minor children engaging in sexual relationships.

2. NAMBLA is highly organized with an internal structure of officers and national and local chapters.

3. Groups solicit membership dues and hold national conferences, like many legal and legitimate organizations, but NAMBLA is secretive.

4. Dues are in the form of child pornography posted to the groups' chat rooms.

— Online sex rings:

1. Rings are loosely organized.

2. Rings consist of people who are members of password-protected chat rooms.

3. Members trade child pornography, discuss strategies for molesting children, and talk about previous sexual assaults on children.

4. Once a member, an individual has access to other members' collections.

5. Reports of intrafamilial child sexual abuse and pornography production entail international participants.

— Pornography as advertising:

1. Images advertise human sexuality limited to the physical and are fairly one-sided.

2. Willingness of profit-oriented companies to spend or invest large amounts of money proves the power of advertising.

3. Collections often have central components of pedophiliac psychology, social orientation, and behavior (Rush, 1981).

4. Children are blackmailed into silence by photographs of themselves engaged in sexual activities arranged by the pedophile.

5. Such pornographic extortion can be accomplished through cellular/mobile phone technology and video iPods, as well as online.

— A significant problem associated with pedophiliac attraction is the process of desensitization and escalation.

1. An increasing level of explicitness or dehumanization may be needed to achieve the same initial thrill.

2. Photos show children being forced into sexual contact, sexually tortured, or worse (Burke et al, 2000).

3. Pornography is shown to potential victims as part of the grooming process, to lower their inhibitions and to show the activity the offender wishes the child to do (Durkin, 1997).

4. Images may be used as trophies (Lanning, 2001).

5. Exposure to pornography may influence offending in an individual who has developed an appetite for sexual deviance, but it is not the sole cause of offending (Marshall, 2000).

— There are 4 classes of offending: downloading, trading, production, and Internet seduction (see also Chapter 2, Victims and Offenders).

1. Categories overlap and revolve around engagement with the Internet and possession of abusive images.

2. Downloading child abuse images is always purposeful and represents a largely passive way to collect images.

   A. Sometimes it involves searching for material, but passive collecting rarely includes substantial direct social engagement with other people engaged in similar activities.

   B. Passive collecting may heighten the justification an individual may feel knowing that others share these interests.

3. Social contact can legitimize and normalize sexual interests.

4. Newness of images ensures status in a trading community.

5. Images may be created according to the personal fantasies of the producers or their perceptions of the market.

6.   Images can also be commissioned by others who express prefer-
     ences for certain types of sexual activities.

PROCESS

— Free samples are often given to attract customers.

— Relatively little is known about the relationship between possession
of abuse images of children and contact offending.

1.   Individuals who produce abuse images commit a contact offense.

2.   Individuals who possess abuse images are less dangerous, not
     always moving from engagement with abuse images to contact
     offending.

3.   The collection of abuse images generates the demand for more
     images, which is met by photographing additional sexual abuse.

— *E-groups* are proprietary chat rooms that users can establish.

1.   The founder or owner of the e-group specifies the level of access
     for others.

2.   Many e-groups exist for trading abuse images of children but
     allow access only to individuals who prove that they are producing
     abusive images.

— Child victims identified in Internet abuse images are usually part of
the offender's real or acquired family or are on the receiving end of a
caregiving relationship.

— Offending may be related to a need to sustain and increase credibility among others, obtain access to desired images of child abuse, and
express sexual behavior.

— Internet relay chat (IRC):

1.   IRC is a more open forum of a similar protocol.

2.   IRC includes newsgroups, a form of bulletin board.

3.   Communication may take place within a few hours, days,
     or weeks, and the same image may appear many times in
     numerous arenas.

4. The people accessing the material can be located anywhere in the world (**Figure 3-2**).

— Information and communication technology (eg, Web cameras, social networking sites, cellular/mobile phones, video iPods) are being used to facilitate pornographic criminal behavior.

EFFECTS

ON USERS OF PORNOGRAPHY

— A common classification scheme describes 4 stages through which users progress after the initial exposure to pornography (Cline, 1994):

1. *Addiction.* The desire and need to keep seeking more images.

2. *Escalation.* The need for more explicit, extreme, and deviant images to obtain the same sexual effect.

3. *Desensitization.* Considering material once viewed as shocking or taboo as acceptable or commonplace.

4. *Acting out.* Performing the behaviors viewed, including exhibitionism; sadism, masochism, or both; rape; or sex with children.

— The body's biological responses contribute to pornography's power.

1. The adrenal hormone epinephrine is released by any emotional stimulus, including pornography.

2. Epinephrine encourages memorization of what is seen as it "rewards" the body with surges of feelings.

3. Memories are subsequently locked into the brain, which explains why people can remember pornographic images seen years before (Cline, 1994).

4. Chemicals called opioids are released by nerve endings in response to pleasure and reinforce the body's desire to repeat the process causing the release.

5. Because these messages often include antisocial attitudes about women, relationships, and behavior, exposure to pornography can be particularly toxic if pornographic images are a child's first exposure to sexuality and no other points of reference exist.

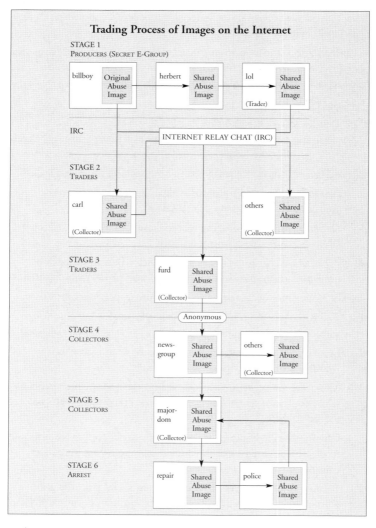

Figure 3-2. The natural history of trading images on the Internet.

DAMAGE TO CHILDREN

— When prematurely exposed to adult pornography, children are thrust into a world they are not prepared to handle.

1.   Adult sexuality involves context and is prepared for incrementally.

2.   Children advance through 4 to 5 stages of cognitive development fairly predictably.

3.   Being exposed to concepts too advanced for their developmental stage can have serious, far-reaching effects.

4.   As children progress through the cognitive stages, they develop morally. If children have a traumatic experience that is beyond their comprehension, it can hinder mental and moral development.

5.   Anecdotal reports of children who have been pornographically exploited reveal significant delayed disclosure, sometimes referred to as *double silencing*.

— It has been suggested that unfettered access to all material, including Internet pornography, helps children develop critical thinking skills. This theory has not proved true (Dorr et al, 1980; Nathanson, 2004; Watkins et al, 1988).

REFERENCES

Burke J, Gentleman A, Willan P. British link to 'snuff' videos. *Guardian Observer*. October 1, 2000. Available at: http://observer.guardian.co.uk/uk_news/story/0,6903,375883.00.htm. Accessed August 27, 2004.

Cline VB. *Pornography's Effects on Adults and Children*. New York, NY: Morality In Media; 1994.

Densen-Gerber J, Hutchinson S. Sexual and commercial exploitation of children: legislative response and treatment challenge. *Child Abuse Negl*. 1979;3:61-66.

Dorr A, Graves SB, Phelps E. Television literacy for young children. *J Commun*. 1980;30(3):71-83.

Durkin KF. Misuse of the Internet by pedophiles: implications for law enforcement and probation practice. *Fed Probat.* 1997;61(3):14-18.

Lanning KV. *Child Molesters: A Behavioral Analysis.* 4th ed. Alexandria, Va: National Center for Missing & Exploited Children; 2001.

Marshall WL. Revisiting the use of pornography by sexual offenders: implications for theory and practice. *J Sex Aggress.* 2000;6:67-77.

Nathanson AI. Factual and evaluative approaches to modifying children's responses to violent television. *J Commun.* 2004;54:321-336.

North American Man/Boy Love Association. Staying safe and happy as a man/boy lover: guidelines developed by NAMBLA activists for surviving in an insane world. *NAMBLA Bulletin.* October, 1991;12(8).

Quayle E, Taylor M. Child pornography and the Internet: perpetuating a cycle of abuse. *Deviant Behav.* 2002;23(4):331-362.

Quayle E, Taylor M. Model of problematic Internet use in people with a sexual interest in children. *Cyberpsychol Behav.* 2003;6(1):93-106.

Rush F. *The Best Kept Secret (Sexual Abuse of Children).* New York, NY: McGraw-Hill; 1981.

Taylor M, Holland G, Quayle E. Typology of paedophile picture collections. *Police Journal.* 2001;74:97-107

Watkins LT, Sprafkin J, Gadow KD, Sadetsky I. Effects of a critical viewing skills curriculum on elementary school children's knowledge and attitudes about television. *J Educ Res.* 1988;31:165-170.

Chapter 4

PROSTITUTION OF CHILDREN

Mary P. Alexander, MA, LPC
James A. H. Farrow, MD, FSAM
Ingrid Leth, Former Senior Adviser, UNICEF
Nancy D. Kellogg, MD
Daniel J. Sheridan, PhD, RN, FAAN
Phyllis L. Thompson, LCSW
Dawn VanPelt, BSN, RN

— *Prostitution of children* is the act of engaging or offering a child's services to perform sexual acts for money or other consideration (**Table 4-1**).

Table 4-1. Factors Contributing to the Prostitution of Children
— The laws primarily target the exploiter and/or pimp but ignore the culpability of the sexual molester and/or john.
— There are predictable situations that make children more at risk to becoming victims of prostitution. Most are runaway, "thrownaway," or deserted children who have experienced sexual abuse, physical abuse, emotional abuse, and/or domestic violence before leaving home. Many become sexually exploited as a result of family dysfunction, familial drug abuse, and recurrent school and other social failures.
— The "infantilization" of prostitution because of the increased demand for "virgins" by molesters and/or johns.
— The laws pertaining to the prostitution of children are not enforced as often or as stringently as they could be.

1. It usually involves extrafamilial *pimps* or female exploiters called *madams.*

2. It also includes familial situations in which parents offer their children to third parties for money or anything of value (called *charm school cases*).

— Prostitution takes many forms: domestic prostituting of children, domestic and international trafficking of children for the purpose of prostitution, or child sex tourism.

— All prostituted children are marginalized, if not alienated, from society.

— Related topics include intimate partner violence and dating violence.

DEFINITIONS

— *Alienation.* A withdrawal or separation of a person from the values of his or her society or family.

— *Marginalization.* Relegation to the outer limits of social standing as a result of alienation; precipitated by psychological and social factors, including childhood abuse and victimization within the family, homelessness, and early onset of serious mental illness (Ringwalt et al, 1998a,b; Sleegers et al, 1998; Widom & Kuhns, 1996).

— *Intimate partner violence (IPV).* Physical, sexual, or psychological harm by a current or former partner or spouse.

1. IPV can occur among heterosexual or homosexual couples.

2. Sexual intimacy is not necessary (Intimate partner violence: overview, 2005).

— *Dating violence.* Violence occurring in a dating relationship wherein an adolescent is the victim or perpetrator.

1. Violence inflicted or sustained in the early dating period often precedes later violence (DeKeseredy & Schwartz, 1994; Gidycz et al, 1993; Himelein, 1995; Lavoie et al, 2000; Malamuth et al, 1995; O'Leary et al, 1994).

2. It is often associated with adolescents' exposure to physical, emotional, and/or sexual domestic violence among parents or friends.

3. Friends are more influential than parents in shaping standards of acceptable dating behaviors during adolescence.

RISK FACTORS

ATTITUDES AND BELIEFS

— Prepubescent and postpubescent children are often included with young women older than 18 years in data on prostitution.

— The prostitution of children is not viewed as a significant problem in Western societies.

1. Children in the sex trade are often regarded as "bad kids" who are to blame for their circumstances (Spangenberg, 2001).

2. Prostitution of children is considered a form of sexual acting out (Hollin & Howells, 1991).

3. Rape myths deny or minimize victim injury or blame victims for their situation.

4. Falsely held beliefs lead to increased victimization of women and escalating violence.

ENVIRONMENTAL FACTORS

— These factors include the presence of a preexisting adult prostitution market.

— Although not all come from situations of neglect, abuse, or poor parental relationships, these aspects are seen in a majority of cases.

— Intrafamilial prostitution is well recognized and may be facilitated through technology.

— The mean age for prostituted boys and girls is 17 years; the average age is 14 years (Klain, 1999; Whitcomb & Eastin, 1998).

— Western societies differ from developing countries, where sexual exploitation occurs at younger ages and has a significant poverty component (Lalor, 1999; UNICEF, 1995).

— Poverty is considered a major force behind the prostitution of children.

— Family dysfunction (eg, violence, mental illness, sexual victimization), familial drug abuse, and recurrent school and social failures are found more often in child sexual exploitation (CSE) cases than poverty (Estes & Weiner, 2001).

— Prostitution of children has been reported in rural communities with methamphetamine home labs.

VICTIM ISSUES

— Most prostituted juveniles in North America are white nonhispanics; the second largest racial group of exploited youths is African American.

— The adolescent developmental task of forming a sexual identity can be negatively impacted by any coercive sexual experiences.

— Child sexual abuse victims are, in their lifetime, 28 times more likely to be arrested for prostitution as compared to children who were not sexually abused (Widom, 1995).

— Homeless or prostituting boys' early, coerced, or negative sexual experiences are more likely to be homosexual than girl's experiences.

1. Early victimization may aggravate the youth's negative self-image and sexual identity confusion (James & Meyerding, 1977).

2. When a questioning male youth hangs out where hustling is prominent, he may be exploring his sexual identity or seeking social acceptance in the gay community (Gonsiorek & Rudolph, 1991; Kruks, 1991). However, most of his sexual experiences will be exploitative, further aggravating a negative self-image.

3. Many young men who are exploited in prostitution in the gay community have difficulty becoming employable and self-sufficient in their 20s.

4. Many remain at considerable risk for human immunodeficiency virus/acquired immunodeficiency syndrome (HIV/AIDS) and substance abuse (Clatts et al, 1998; Gleghorn et al, 1998; Luna, 1997).

INFANTILIZATION OF PROSTITUTION
— Increases because of the risk of contracting AIDS.

— There is a high demand for virgins.

— Molesters and *johns*, the term for males who solicit prostituted people, believe that "virgins" (prepubescent children) will not have sexually transmitted diseases (STDs) since they have not been exposed through prior sexual intercourse.

— Some abusers believe that having sex with a virgin cures STDs.

— Prostituted children usually have been sexually abused and exploited by their parent(s), a pimp, or others long before they became prostituted.

— Prepubescent children are at high risk for AIDS and STDs because of the likelihood of anal or vaginal tearing during intercourse.

EFFECTS

CONSEQUENCES OF SEXUAL EXPLOITATION
— Youths involved in prostitution have a significant increase in medical and psychosocial consequences compared to those not involved.

— Other results:

1. Dropping out of school at an earlier age

2. Having fewer constructive hobbies and less sports participation

3. Developing depression, posttraumatic stress disorder (PTSD), drug abuse, and other symptoms of psychological distress (Rohde et al, 2001; Smart & Walsh, 1993)

4. Coerced substance abuse is a well-recognized further impact on victims; the most common drugs of choice are methamphetamine and cocaine.

5. High incidence of pregnancy among young women (Deisher et al, 1989; Greene & Ringwalt, 1998)

6. The leading cause of death in prostituted children is murder; the second leading cause is HIV/AIDS.

CONSEQUENCES OF DATING VIOLENCE

— Acquaintance rape occurs in 19% to 53% of adolescent dating relationships (Gray & Foshee, 1997).

— Direct physical and psychological violence against an adolescent can cause lifelong negative health consequences; psychological violence has additional impact, whether the adolescent is a direct victim or a witness of physical violence against others.

— Early detection of abuse and treatment leads to better outcomes (American Academy of Pediatrics, Committee on Child Abuse and Neglect, 1991).

— Injuries range from minor to life-threatening.

— Pregnancy can result from IPV and represents a time of increased risk for escalating violence.

— More sexually transmitted infections (STIs) and urinary tract infections occur in abused women, especially those experiencing sexual violence (Glass et al, 2003).

— Sexual abuse is present in 50% of women and 23% of men receiving psychiatric help (Ainscough & Toon, 1993).

— Childhood sexual abuse is linked to adult psychological problems (eg, anxiety, anger, depression, revictimization, self-mutilation/self-harm, sexual problems, substance abuse, suicidality, impaired self-concept, interpersonal problems, obsessions and compulsions, dissociation, PTSD, and somatization).

— Poor concepts of self-care can also develop.

— Victim violence:

1. Repeated exposure to violence, even if not directed toward the adolescent, can lead to a propensity to commit violent acts.

2. The adolescent perpetrates violence as a learned behavior from childhood.

3. Adolescents in the juvenile justice system must be examined in a

context beyond the assault to determine appropriate intervention and treatment (Salter et al, 2003).

INTERACTIONS WITH SOCIAL SERVICES AND HEALTHCARE PROFESSIONALS

— Interactions can be challenging because these youths are suspicious of adults' motives based on past manipulation and exploitation by adults and experiences with the juvenile justice system.

— Transient and often violent lifestyles, dependence on drugs, and the need to drop out of sight further isolate them.

— Young women are often denied access to helpful professionals by a controlling adult figure, usually a pimp, abusive boyfriend, or adult relative (Deisher et al, 1989).

— Victims may enter the healthcare setting with medical or psychiatric problems related to victimization.

— Victims may enter after suffering physical or sexual assault injuries, leading to disclosure of the abusive experiences.

— They may be brought to a healthcare setting after pornographic materials are found or the perpetrator confesses.

— Once a child or adolescent is identified as a victim of abuse, protocols for physical and sexual abuse are employed and the police and child protective services (CPS) agencies are notified (see Chapters 3, Child Pornography, 8, Principles of Investigation, 11, Investigating Cyber-Enticement, and 14, Legal Approaches to Internet Cases).

— Types of help sought by prostituted adolescents:

1. Pregnancy testing
2. Treatment of STIs
3. Abortion services
4. Treatment for miscarriage
5. Drug overdose interventions
6. Treatment of abscesses, especially at injection sites

— Trauma presentations:

1. Facial bruising and lacerations

2. Bruised and broken ribs

3. Vaginal and rectal tears

4. Bruising to abdomen and back

5. Cut and stab wounds

6. Gunshots

NOTE: Any of these presentations should immediately be a red flag for abuse screening.

INTERVENTIONS

— Few providers or programs address all of a victim's needs.

— Treatment is often fragmented.

1. It usually does not address safety, education, social and trade skills, or protection.

2. Short-term therapy or treatment rarely addresses sexual victimization; the problem is compounded by victims' reluctance to disclose abuse and tendency to avoid treatment until severe problems with physical and mental health occur.

— Reasons why victims do not want help or are afraid to seek and/or accept help include:

1. Extensive grooming to accommodate victimization.

2. Threats, blackmail, beatings, mutilation, and torture by pimps or perpetrators.

3. Fear of being reported to juvenile justice system, being placed in foster care, or having to return to dysfunctional or abusive family (Unger et al, 1998).

— To avoid disclosure and discovery, children and adolescents often lie about age and circumstances.

— If service providers try to gather information leading to police or CPS intervention, victims may recant, refuse services, and leave.

REFERENCES

Ainscough C, Toon K. *Breaking Free: Help for Survivors of Child Sexual Abuse*. London, England: Sheldon Press; 1993.

American Academy of Pediatrics, Committee on Child Abuse and Neglect. Guidelines for the evaluation of sexual abuse of children. *Pediatrics*. 1991;87:254-260.

Clatts MC, Davis WR, Sotheran JL, Atillasoy A. Correlates and distribution of HIV risk behaviors among homeless youths in New York City: implications for prevention and policy. *Child Welfare*. 1998;77(2):195-207.

Deisher RW, Farrow JA, Hope K, Litchfield C. The pregnant adolescent prostitute. *Am J Dis Child*. 1989;143:1162-1165.

DeKeseredy WS, Schwartz MD. Locating a history of some Canadian woman abuse in elementary and high school dating relationships. *Humanity Soc*. 1994;18:43-63.

Estes RJ, Weiner HA. *The Commercial Sexual Exploitation of Children in the US, Canada and Mexico*. Philadelphia, Penn: University of Pennsylvania, School of Social Work; 2001.

Gidycz CA, Coble C, Latham L, Layman MJ. Sexual assault experience in adulthood and prior victimization experiences. *Psychol Women Q*. 1993;17:151-168.

Glass NE, Campbell JC, Kub J, Sharps PW, Fredland N, Yonas M. Adolescent dating violence: prevalence, risk factors, health outcomes, and implications for clinical practice. *J Obstet Gynecol Neonatal Nurs*. 2003;32:2-12.

Gleghorn AA, Marx R, Vittinghoff E, Katz MH. Association between drug use patterns and HIV risks among homeless, runaway, and street youths in Northern California. *Drug Alcohol Depend*. 1998;51(3):219-227.

Gonsiorek JC, Rudolph JR. Homosexual identity: coming out and other developmental events. In: Gonsiorek J, Weinrich J, eds.

Homosexuality: Research Implications for Public Policy. Newbury Park, Calif: Sage Publications: 1991;161-176.

Gray H, Foshee VA. Adolescent dating violence: differences between one-sided and mutually violent profiles. *J Interpers Violence*. 1997; 12:126-141.

Greene JM, Ringwalt CL. Pregnancy among three national samples of runaway and homeless youth. *J Adolesc Health*. 1998;23(6):370-377.

Himelein MJ. Risk factors for sexual victimization in dating: a longitudinal study of college women. *Psychol Women Q*. 1995;19:31-48.

Hollin CR, Howells K, eds. *Clinical Approaches to Sex Offenders and Their Victims*. New York, NY: John Wiley and Sons; 1991.

Intimate partner violence: overview. Centers for Disease Control and Prevention Web site. Available at: http://www.cdc.gov/ncipc/fact sheets/ipvoverview.htm. Accessed February 9, 2005.

James J, Meyerding J. Early sexual experiences as a factor in prostitution. *Arch Sex Behav*. 1977;1:31-42.

Klain EJ. *Prostitution of Children and Child-Sex Tourism: An Analysis of Domestic and International Responses*. Alexandria, VA: National Center for Missing and Exploited Children; 1999.

Kruks G. Gay and lesbian homeless/street youth: special issues and concerns. *J Adoles Health*. 1991;12(7):515-518.

Lalor KJ. Street children: a comparative perspective. *Child Abuse Negl*. 1999;23(8):759-770.

Lavoie F, Robitaille L, Hebert M. Teen dating relationships and aggression. *Violence Against Women*. 2000;6:6-36.

Luna GC. *Youths Living with HIV: Self-Evident Truths*. New York, NY: Harrington Park Press; 1997.

Malamuth NM, Linz D, Heavey CL, Barnes G, Acker M. Using the confluence of sexual aggression to predict men's conflicts with women: a 10-year follow-up study. *J Pers Soc Psychol*. 1995;60:353-369.

O'Leary KD, Malone J, Tyree A. Physical aggression in early marriage: prerelationship and relationship effects. *J Consult Clin Psychol*. 1994; 62:594-602.

Ringwalt CL, Greene JM, Robertson MJ. Familial backgrounds and risk behaviors of youth with thrownaway experiences. *J Adolesc*. 1998a; 21(3):241-252.

Ringwalt CL, Greene JM, Robertson MJ, McPheeters M. The prevalence of homelessness among adolescents in the United States. *Am J Public Health*. 1998b;88(9):1325-1329.

Rohde P, Noell J, Ochs L, Seeley JR. Depression, suicidal ideation and STD-related risk in homeless older adolescents. *J Adolesc*. 2001; 24(4): 447-460.

Salter D, McMillan D, Richards M, et al. Development of sexually abusive behavior in sexually victimized males: a longitudinal study. *Lancet*. 2003;361:471-476.

Sleegers J, Spijker J, van Limbeek J, van Engeland H. Mental health problems among homeless adolescents. *Acta Psychiatr Scand*. 1998; 97(4):253-259.

Smart FG, Walsh GW. Predictors of depression in street youth. *Adolescence*. 1993;28(109):41-53.

Spangenberg M. Prostituted youth in New York City: an overview. ECPAT-USA. 2001. Available at: http://www.ecpatusa.org/pdf/cseypnc.pdf. Accessed August 21, 2003.

Unger JB, Simon TR, Newman TL, Montgomery SB, Kipke MD, Albornoz M. Early adolescent street youth: an overlooked population with unique problems and service needs. *J Early Adolesc*. 1998; 18(4): 325-349.

UNICEF. The Convention on the Rights of the Child. London, England: UK Committee for UNICEF; 1995.

Whitcomb D, Eastin J. *Joining Forces Against Child Sexual Exploitation: Models for a Multijurisdictional Team Approach*. Washington, DC: Office for Victims of Crime, US Dept of Justice; 1998.

Widom CS, Kuhns JB. Childhood victimization and subsequent risk for promiscuity, prostitution, and teenage pregnancy: a prospective study. *Am J Public Health.* 1996;86(11):1607-1612.

Widom CS. *Victims of Childhood Sexual Abuse: Later Criminal Consequences.* Washington, DC: National Institute of Justice, US Dept of Justice; 1995. NCJ 151525.

Chapter 5

CYBER-ENTICEMENT AND INTERNET TRAVELERS

Jeffrey A. Dort, JD
David Finkelhor, PhD
Terry Jones, BA (Hons), PGCE
L. Alvin Malesky, Jr, PhD
Kimberly Mitchell, PhD
Janis Wolak, JD

BACKGROUND INFORMATION

— Concerns about Internet usage:

1. Cyber addictions, where individuals spend an inordinate amount of time online (Brody, 2000; Cooper et al, 2000; Putnam & Maheu, 2000)

2. Online infidelity, where online usage causes relationship and marital discord (Young et al, 2000)

3. Advancement of extremist ideologies (eg, racism) (Schafer, 2002)

4. Criminal activity (Conly, 1989)

— Internet pedophilia has developed as a result of social, psychological, and physical issues.

— The Internet allows pedophiles to effortlessly circulate all types of material; the actual images being circulated of children are indecent and abusive.

— The real faces of abuse victims are available in a wide-open forum, constantly recirculating and continually revictimizing, with no prospect of deletion or closure for the victims.

— Previously, pedophiles who photographed children had to devise a way to surreptitiously develop or reproduce the illegal pictures. The Internet and digital photography have eliminated those barriers.

1. Child abuse images can be instantaneously recorded, stored, and distributed with ease.

2. Most child abuse material circulating on the Internet is not commercially driven or controlled.

3. Recent images are set in domestic surroundings with increasingly younger victims being subjected to more violence (Taylor, 2003).

4. Members of organized crime groups have become interested in the commercial aspects of pedophilia, particularly Web-based pedophilia (National Criminal Intelligence Service, 2003).

— Millions of homes in the United States have Internet access (US Department of Commerce [USDOC], 2001).

— Finkelhor et al (2000) found:

1. 20% of children received an online sexual solicitation.

2. 1 in 33 received an "aggressive sexual solicitation."

3. 25% told parents when they had been sexually solicited.

4. 25% had unwanted exposures to Internet images of unclothed people or people having sex.

5. 97% of sexual solicitations were made by people the child victims had originally met online.

6. Many children reported that the people wanted them to engage in cybersex.

— Internet access is available at various public venues (eg, libraries, universities, cyber coffee shops).

— Relatively few families or young people take action against the negative aspects of the Internet.

— Why the Internet is used for sexual gratification (Cooper, 1998):

1. Accessibility

2. Affordability

3. Anonymity

— Virtually any sexual material ranging from soft-core pornography to extreme pictures and video clips of bestiality, torture, and pedophilia can be found and accessed online (Durkin, 1997; Durkin & Bryant, 1995; Garreau, 1993; Kim & Bailey, 1997; Leiblum, 1997).

— A large number of images and even video clips depicting pornography can be acquired at relatively no cost.

— The Internet is an ideal tool to engage in sexual behavior (especially illegal sexual behavior) when individuals want to conceal their identities. The anonymity of the Internet permits individuals to hide or misrepresent themselves and to assume multiple online personas and identities.

— Cellular/mobile phone technology and Web cameras are other venues of exploitation particularly associated with compliant victimization.

— Adolescent brain development is incomplete until well past the end of the second decade of life. The prefrontal cortex is the last part of the brain to fully mature, and it is this area that controls judgment, impulses, and emotional behaviors. Cyberawareness is a complex phenomenon that, in the absence of real world personal contacts, can be problematic for youths who untimately make poor decisions regarding their online activities (Berson, 2003).

SCOPE
— A key component of Internet pedophilia is local, yet the posted images are instantaneously global.

1. Worldwide, pedophiles view, collect, and use child abuse images for sexual arousal (global problem).

2. The same individuals are likely to be a risk to children in the neighborhood (local problem).

3. Proactive identification of such individuals locally is difficult and normally requires national or international police tactics.

— Little is known about the relationship between physical child molestation and photographing such abuse.

DEFINITIONS

— *Aggressive solicitations.* Suspect asks child to meet, calls child on the phone, or sends child regular mail, money, or gifts. Most are ended by logging off the computer, leaving the site, and/or blocking the person.

— *Chat rooms.* Sites on the Internet where individuals communicate in real time by typing text. Chat rooms cater to various interests and age groups.

— *Cybersex.* A form of fantasy sex that involves interactive chat room sessions during which the participants describe sexual acts and sometimes disrobe and masturbate.

— *E-mail.* Abbreviation of electronic mail. E-mail is the most commonly used facet of the Internet (USDOC, 2001).

— *Habituation.* A term used to describe a decreased sexual responsiveness to repeated visual exposure. Most individuals who download images of child pornography do so for sexual arousal (Quayle & Taylor, 2002). However, they tire of viewing and masturbating to the same set of images and continually search for more stimulating/arousing material to fuel their sexual fantasies. Desire for novel material is one of the mechanisms that drives the production of child pornography.

— *Hyperlinks.* Means of accessing other Web sites simply by clicking on a certain word, phrase, or picture.

— *Newsgroups.* Sites on the Internet where electronic messages on the same general topic are collected. Once a message is read, the reader can respond to the "post" publicly (so the entire newsgroup can read response) or privately.

— *Proactive approach.* Officers initiate an investigation of the problem area rather than of a specific crime and then wait for the perpetrator to contact them.

— *Reactive approach.* Victims report crimes to police, then officers respond to information provided before an investigation is initiated; these cases are more typical in police work.

— *Remailers.* Programs that strip header information from e-mails (Kopelev, 1999), electronic encryption software (Cusack, 1996), and passwords (Nordland & Bartholet, 2001) to help conceal identities.

— *Traveler.* In Internet sexual exploitation cases, a person who contacts a child younger than 18 years on the Internet and then attempts to meet the child to engage in sexual activities (Freeh, 1998); scenarios can lead to violent sexual crimes and murder (Freeh, 1998). Traveler variations include:

1. *Local travelers.* Stay in the town or area where they reside and travel a short distance (fewer than 50 miles, for example) to meet intended child victims (Wolak et al, 2003b). They limit their victim search to a specific state or region or only target chat rooms with a location as part of its name. By staying near home, local travelers feel more in control.

2. *Interstate or intrastate travelers.* Journey more than 50 miles out of or within state (M Harmony, oral communication, March 2004). They risk more, travel further, and break more laws than local travelers. Federal law prohibits interstate travel with the intent of engaging in a sexual act with a minor. The distance traveled is often used by prosecutors to argue the crime was premeditated and deliberate, and it solidifies the intent element required by statute.

3. *Global travelers.* Go to other countries to engage in sexual acts with children. The media uses the term ***sex tourist***. They plan and prepare more than any other type of traveler and are sometimes part of tour groups centered around sex (Sex "tourist" gets seven years, 2000; Robson, 2004). American citizens can be arrested for sex crimes they commit while traveling overseas.

4. *Victim travelers.* Set up sex meetings and convince and pay for children to travel to their location (eg, Levesque, 2000); a rare traveler variation. Victims appear to be willing participants, but

the offenders use the lure of sex or money to convince the children to travel. Law defines these children as victims. Most federal and state laws do not distinguish between *who* is doing the actual traveling, concentrating on whether the purpose is to bring 2 parties together for sexual purposes (eg, 18 USC § 2423(b) 2003).

5. *Traveler no-shows.* Do not show up at the selected meeting location even after months of communications with victim; another rare traveler variation. This occurs for various reasons, including (1) travelers get worried and frightened of being caught, (2) travelers discover the meeting is a sting operation, (3) travelers realize meeting is illegal, and (4) travelers never intended to show up. Regardless of motive and the fact that no travel has taken place, traveler no-show incidents are important—travelers can take months and even years to coordinate a successful meeting, so some failed meetings must be expected (Nurenberg, 2002).

6. *Sting operations.* Police officers pose as children in undercover operations online. They involve some travel, but no children. Adults begin conversations with the officers posing as children and sometimes proposition or entice them to meet for sex. The officers set up the meeting and arrange a location. When the adult arrives, no child is there. The suspect is arrested for attempting to meet a child for sexual purposes. Sting operations can involve any of the preceding 5 categories.

— *Traveling.* Crossing state lines to engage a minor in sex.

— *Web sites.* Electronic locations on the World Wide Web that often comprise multiple Web pages. They are essentially computer files encoded in hypertext markup language that can be accessed by Internet users.

RISK FACTORS

— Many children who begin online relationships with abusers fit a particular profile (Wolak et al, 2003a). They:

1. Are searching for anyone who will listen to them.

2. Have a greater tendency for conflict or lack of communication with their parents.

3. Have high levels of delinquency, including committing assault, vandalism, and theft.

4. Possess a troubled personality due to depression, peer victimization, or a distressing life event.

— Some youths willingly leave their homes and become compliant victims (Wolak et al, 2004).

— Youths at risk tend to be older (aged 14 to 17 years), female, troubled, have high rates of Internet use, use chat rooms, talk with strangers online, engage in high-risk online behavior, and use the Internet in households other than their own (Mitchell et al, 2001).

— A high level of technical sophistication does not necessarily equate a greater risk to children.

— Current assessment procedures cannot determine an individual's risk for contact offenses based solely on online behavior.

— Sexual gratification is not the sole motivation for collecting Internet child pornography (O'Connell & Taylor, 1998; Quayle & Taylor, 2002a).

1. Images are often part of a larger collection or series supposedly named after the victim in the pictures (Lee, 2003).

2. Offenders may attempt to complete an entire series, like a baseball card collector.

3. Requests for specific images are routinely made on pedophile bulletin boards (Lee, 2003).

4. Collectors may exchange images to increase social status and credibility in virtual pedophile communities (O'Connell & Taylor, 1998).

5. Some collect images of child pornography that are not sexually arousing with the intent of helping others complete a series.

6. *Collector syndrome* refers to the compulsive acquisition of pictures

for their own sake, rather than for a discriminating collection (Taylor, 1999).

— The Internet may introduce deviant fantasies to individuals who may not have previously explored them, but this is speculative.

1. A person who would never approach a child in the real world may make such contact in cyberspace just to see what happens.

2. If these individuals begin masturbating while interacting with children (or adults they believe are children) online, it is likely that their deviant sexual fantasies will be further reinforced.

3. The physical reinforcement associated with masturbation plus the cognitive distortions introduced and subsequently strengthened through online interactions may move individuals closer to actually offending against a child than if they had never accessed the Internet.

INTERNET COMPONENTS USED FOR SEXUALLY DEVIANT AND ILLEGAL ACTIVITY

— Newsgroups, e-mail, Web sites, and chat rooms can be employed for sexually deviant and/or illegal purposes (Kim & Bailey, 1997).

— Uses:

1. Trafficking child pornography (Huycke, 1997; Kantrowitz et al, 1994; Thompson, 2002)

2. Locating children to molest (Armagh, 1998; Booth, 1999; Durkin & Bryant, 1995; Jackson, 1989; Levy et al, 1995; McLaughlin, 2000)

3. Assisting in communication between pedophiles (Durkin, 1997; Kopelev, 1999)

NEWSGROUPS

— Provide peer support to individuals struggling with pedophilic desires as well as validation of pedophilic urges (Armagh, 1998; Durkin, 1997).

— Disseminate information.

— Consolidate and bring together individuals with similar deviant interests.

— Provide support for deviant and illegal sexual desires and activities.

E-Mail

— E-mail allows for rapid and inexpensive correspondence by transmitting electronic messages from one computer to another over the Internet.

— Still images, video clips, and audio clips can be sent as attachments in e-mail or in the body of the message itself.

Web Sites

— Provide information on numerous subjects using photographs, video clips, text, sound clips, and even live images.

— Directly facilitate the victimization of children.

— Are used to advance ideology of propedophile groups.

— Include hyperlinks to legitimate child organizations on Web sites.

Chat Rooms

— The anonymity of cyberspace makes it difficult to discern if an individual is a child communicating with other children for benign reasons or an adult masquerading as a child for nefarious purposes.

— Some advocate the sexual exploitation of children.

— These forums bring pedophiles together and act as a consolidating mechanism to facilitate the exchange of child pornography and to reinforce deviant views pertaining to adult/minor sexual contact (US Department of Justice, Equality and Law Reform, 1998).

Web Cameras, Mobile Phone Technology, and Social Networking Sites

— These forms of communication may afford real time transmission of images between a compliant victim and an offender.

— Autoerotic exhibitionism is common with use of Web cams, and offenders diminish barriers by exposing themselves first in the contacts with youths.

— Mobile phones allow pictures, text messaging, and image transmissions between victims and offenders.

— Social networking sites allow millions of youths to invite others to be their "friends," at times including offenders who use this popular online contact to groom potential victims.

PROCESS

— The practice of gathering child erotica is underreported.

— Suspects often seek out and save decent images of children as well as illegal material.

LOCATING CHILDREN TO MOLEST

— Most offenders know their victims before offending.

— Online chat rooms appear to be a common forum used by offenders to contact potential victims (Armagh, 1998; Kantrowitz et al, 1994; Kopelev, 1999; Lamb, 1998; McLaughlin, 2000; Thomas, 1997).

— After establishing contact, offenders attempt to set up an in-person meeting with their potential victims.

INTERNET'S ROLE IN THE ETIOLOGY OF CHILD SEXUAL ABUSE

— If individuals spend much time interacting in propedophilic chat rooms, visiting propedophilic Web sites, and communicating with individuals advocating for the sexual exploitation of minors, the behaviors and attitudes observed are likely to be adopted and/or reinforced.

— Modeling or observing others can serve a disinhibitory function and effect changes in moral judgment.

IMAGE ANALYSIS

— False images of child abuse (***pseudo images***) exist, but in relatively low numbers.

— They are created by manually or digitally replacing the heads on adult pornographic images with those of children (***morphing***).

1. Adult features can be altered to present a more childlike body image.

2. Limited examples of generating fake images using computer software have appeared. Whether the material is old or new, almost all the victims in child abuse images are real children.

— The following questions must be answered in the victim identification process:

1. Who is the child?

2. Where is the child?

3. When was the image created?

4. Has the child been found?

5. Who should investigate the crime?

— The Internet is used to collect/trade child pornography.

1. The Internet allows for the rapid and inexpensive reproduction and exchange of these images.

2. It fosters a sense of cognitive dissonance where individuals do not believe they are doing anything wrong or are harming anyone by simply downloading these images from the Web.

3. Downloading child pornography perpetuates child sexual abuse on multiple levels.

— Text-based child abuse accounts or fantasy stories are widely used by suspects to stimulate sexual arousal.

— There is a relationship between downloading online child pornography and committing contact sex offenses.

1. Sex offenders convicted of possession of child pornography or traveling charges commit contact sexual offenses at a higher rate (30.5 victims per offender) than sex offenders convicted specifically of contact sex crimes (9.6 victims per offender) (Hernandez, 2000).

2. Many adjudicated Internet offenders have at least as many contact victims as individuals convicted of contact sex crimes.

REFERENCES

Armagh G. A safety net for the Internet: protecting our children. *Juvenile Justice*. 1998;5(1):9-15.

Berson IR. Making the connection between brain processing and cyberawareness: a developmental reality. Paper presented at: proceedings of Netsafe II, Society, Safety, and the Internet Symposium; July 9, 2003; Auckland, New Zealand.

Booth W. Internet target: sexual predators. *Washington Post*. December 7, 1999:A29.

Brody JE. Cybersex gives birth to a psychological disorder. *New York Times*. May 16, 2000:7, 12.

Conly CH. *Organizing for Computer Crime Investigation and Prosecution*. Washington, DC: US Dept of Justice; 1989.

Cooper A. Sexuality and the Internet: surfing into the new millennium. *Cyberpsychol Behav*. 1998;1(2):187-193.

Cooper A, Delmonico DL, Burg R. Cybersex users, abusers, and compulsives: new findings and implications. *Sex Addict Compulsivity*. 2000;7:5-29.

Cusack J. The murky world of Internet porn: the 'Orchid Club' shakes up the law. *World Press Review*. 1996;43:8-10.

Durkin KF. Misuse of the Internet by pedophiles: implications for law enforcement and probation practice. *Fed Probat*. 1997;61(3):14-18.

Durkin KF, Bryant CD. Log on to sex: some notes on the carnal computer and erotic cyberspace as an emerging research frontier. *Deviant Behav*. 1995;16(3):179-200.

18 USC § 2423(b) (2003).

Finkelhor D, Mitchell KJ, Wolak J. *Online Victimization: A Report on the Nation's Youth*. Alexandria, Va: National Center for Missing & Exploited Children; 2000.

Freeh L. Child pornography on the Internet and the sexual exploitation of children. Speech presented at: Senate Appropriations Subcommittee for the Departments of Commerce, Justice, and State, the Judiciary, and Related Agencies; March 10, 1998; Washington, DC. Available at: http://www.eff.org/Censorship/Internet_censorship_bills/1998/19980310_freeh_allen_sen_cjs_app.testimony. Accessed November 29, 2004.

Garreau J. Bawdy bytes: the growing world of cybersex. *Washington Post*. November 29, 1993:A1, A10.

Hernandez AE. Self-reported contact sexual offenses by participants in the Federal Bureau of Prisons' sex offender treatment program: implications for Internet sex offenders. Poster session presented at: 19th Annual Research and Treatment Conference of the Association for the Treatment of Sexual Abusers; November, 2000; San Diego, Calif.

Huycke DF. Protecting our children: the US customs service child pornography enforcement program. *The Police Chief*. 1997;34:34-35.

Jackson RL. Child molesters use electronic networks: computer-crime sleuths go undercover. *Los Angeles Times*. October 1, 1989:20, 21.

Kantrowitz B, King P, Rosenberg D. Child abuse in cyberspace. *Newsweek*. April 18, 1994:40.

Kim PY, Bailey JM. Sidestreets on the information highway: paraphilias and sexual variations on the Internet. *J Sex Educ Ther*. 1997; 22(1):35-43.

Kopelev SD. Cyber sex offenders: how to proactively investigate Internet crimes against children. *Law Enforcement Technology*. 1999; 26(11):46-50.

Lamb M. Cybersex: research notes on the characteristics of the visitors to online chat rooms. *Deviant Behav*. 1998;19:121-135.

Lee J. High tech helps child pornographers and their pursuers. *New York Times* [electronic version]. February, 2003. Available at: http://www.nytimes.com/2003/02/09technology/09PORN.html. Accessed February 9, 2003.

Leiblum SR. Sex and the Net: clinical implications. *J Sex Educ Ther*. 1997;22(1):21-27.

Levesque WR. 71 years to punish man's affair with teen. *St. Petersburg Times*. May 27, 2000. Available at: http://www.sptimes.com/News/ 052700/TampaBay/71_years_to_punish_ma.shtml. Accessed February 1, 2004.

Levy S, Hafner K, Rosenstiel T, et al. No place for kids? *Newsweek*. July 3, 1995:47-50.

McLaughlin JF. Cyber child sex offender typology. Available at: http: //www.ci.keene.nh.us/police/Typology.htm. Accessed June 15, 2000.

Mitchell KJ, Finkelhor D, Wolak J. Risk factors for and impact of online sexual solicitation of youth. *JAMA*. 2001;285:3011-3014.

National Criminal Intelligence Service. Sex offences against children, including online abuse. In: *United Kingdom Threat Assessment of Serious and Organised Crime 2003*. London, England: National Criminal Intelligence Service; 2003. Available at: http://ncis.gov.uk/ ukta/2003/threat09.asp. Accessed January 5, 2005.

Nordland R, Bartholet J. The web's dark secret. *Newsweek*. March 19, 2001:44-51.

Nurenberg G. Cracking down on online predators. G4techTV Web site. August 22, 2002. Available at: http://www.techtv.com/news/ internet/story/0,24195,3397013,00.html. Accessed January 27, 2004.

O'Connell R, Taylor M. Paedophile networks on the Internet: the evidential implications of paedophile picture posting on the Internet. Paper presented at: Combating Paedophile Information Networks in Europe (COPINE) Project Conference; January, 1998; Dublin Castle, Ireland.

Putnam DE, Maheu MM. Online sexual addiction and compulsivity: integrating web resources and behavioral telehealth in treatment. *Sex Addict Compulsivity*. 2000;7:91-112.

Quayle E, Taylor M. Child pornography and the Internet: perpetuating a cycle of abuse. *Deviant Behav*. 2002;23(4):331-362.

Robson S. S. Korea base museum director arrested in Arkansas porn sting. *Stars and Stripes*. European ed. January 10, 2004. Available at: http://www.estripes.com/article.asp?section=104&article+18977&archive=true. Accessed February 1, 2004.

Schafer JA. Spinning the web of hate: web-based hate propagation by extremist organizations. *J Crim Justice Pop Cult*. 2002;9(2):69-88.

Sex "tourist" gets seven years. BBC News Web site. October 20, 2000. Available at: http://news.bbc.co.uk/1/hi/world/europe/980337.stm. Accessed February 1, 2004.

Taylor M. The nature and dimensions of child pornography on the Internet. Paper presented at: International Conference Combating Child Pornography on the Internet; September, 1999; Vienna, Austria.

Taylor M. Victim identification project. Presented at: COPINE Presentation to European Parliament; December, 2003; Brussels, Belgium.

Thomas DS. Cyberspace pornography: problems with enforcement. *Internet Res: Electron Networking Appl Policy*. 1997;7(3):201-207.

Thompson CW. FBI cracks child porn ring based on Internet. *Washington Post*. March 19, 2002:A2.

US Department of Commerce. *Home Computers and Internet Use in the United States: August 2000*. Washington, DC: Government Printing Office; September, 2001. P23-207.

US Department of Justice, Equality and Law Reform. *Illegal and Harmful Use of the Internet*. Dublin, Ireland: The Stationery Office; 1998.

Wolak J, Finkelhor D, Mitchell K. Internet-initiated sex crimes against minors: implications for prevention based findings from a national study. *J Adolesc Health*. 2004;35:424.e11-424.e20.

Wolak J, Mitchell KJ, Finkelhor D. Escaping or connecting? Characteristics of youth who form close online relationships. *J Adolesc*. 2003a;26:105-119.

Wolak J, Mitchell KJ, Finkelhor D. *Internet Sex Crimes Against Minors: The Response of Law Enforcement*. Alexandria, Va: National Center for Missing & Exploited Children; 2003b.

Young KS, Griffin-Shelley E, Cooper A, O'Mara J, Buchanan J. Online infidelity: a new dimension in couple relationships with implications for evaluation and treatment. *Sex Addict Compulsivity*. 2000;7:59-64.

Chapter 6

SEX TOURISM AND HUMAN TRAFFICKING

Elena Azaola, PhD
Sharon W. Cooper, MD, FAAP
Richard J. Estes, DSW, ACSW
Sp Agt Donald B. Henley
Nicole G. Ives, MSW, PhD (Candidate)
Sp Agt Eileen R. Jacob
Bernadette McMenamin, AO
Daniel J. Sheridan, PhD, RN, FAAN
Dawn Van Pelt, BSN, RN
Bharathi A. Venktraman, Esq
Neil Alan Weiner, PhD

DEFINITIONS

— *Trafficking.* "[T]he transport, harboring, or sale of persons within national or across international borders through coercion, force, kidnapping, deception or fraud, for purposes of placing persons in situations of forced labor or services, such as forced prostitution, domestic servitude, debt bondage, or other slavery-like practices" (18 USC § 1589 et seq). International trafficking in human beings is one aspect of the commercial sexual exploitation of children (CSEC) and youths.

— *Domestic trafficking of children.* Trafficking of citizens or permanent residents of a nation within their own country.

— *Child sex tourism.* Travel, usually across international borders, with the intention of engaging in a commercial sex act with a child. It develops in response to the demand by locals as well as foreigners for children as sexual objects.

BACKGROUND INFORMATION

— About 600 000 to 800 000 people worldwide are trafficked across international borders annually; 14 000 to 18 000 of these victims are trafficked to the United States (US Department of State [USDOS], 2004).

— Some estimate that up to 1 million people are trafficked annually within or across national borders (deBaca & Tisi, 2002).

— Globalization is the major force behind the rapid international increase and expansion of the child sex trade. The interconnectedness of economies, technologies, and communities opens access to vulnerable children.

— The United States is cracking down on child sexual abuse by enacting stronger laws, increasing law enforcement efforts, tightening employment screening measures, conducting police checks, and compiling and maintaining sex offender databases to track offenders. As a result, sex offenders are traveling outside of this country and other countries with these increased legal approaches to destinations where they are unknown.

— The causal factors are multiple, interrelated, and complex, with poverty the catalyst.

— Exploiters include pimps, traffickers, corrupt authorities, lax law enforcement officers, and child sex abusers.

— Unlike trafficking in drugs or arms, human trafficking requires no movement, no selling, and no mass shipment.

1. Force, fraud, coercion, or other threatened harm can be used to overwhelm the victim's will to resist and convince the victim to perform the labor or services demanded.

2. Many trafficking victims are foreign-born, but a victim can be born, live, and enslaved in a single location.

— Various means are employed to break the will of the victim.

1. This may involve the abuse of young women from Eastern Europe for commercial sex, child domestic workers from Western Africa for household labor, East Asian sweatshop workers to manufacture garments, or African American agricultural workers for harvesting crops.

2. Exploiters may use physical and emotional abuse, rape, and torture (Aghatise, 2004).

3. Victims may become ensnared in organized crime rings that convince families to send their daughters to countries with the promise of marriage and a rich life.

— Instead of calling it trafficking, professional buyers and entrepreneurs of the sex industry call it "voluntary migration for sex work" (Raymond, 2004).

— Its existence may be minimized or actually denied by countries that fear the loss of tourism money.

1. Few real data exist to validate the sex crimes, especially those against children.

2. Western governments can deny the involvement of their nationals in child sex tourism because they have no reference database to prove it exists.

— Historical practices and local abusers contribute to the sexual demand for children.

— Recently, foreign tourists, military personnel, and businessmen have significantly increased the demand for prostituted children.

OFFENDERS

— Persons who benefit financially from national and international trafficking of children for sexual purposes:

1. Amateur traffickers

2. Small groups of organized criminals

3. Multilayered trafficking networks that are organized both nationally and internationally (Graycar, 1999; Lederer, 2001; Richard, 1999; Scholenhardt, 1999; US Department of State [USDOS], 2003; Yoon, 1997)

— Large networks of trafficking "functionaries" are needed (see also **Table 2-11** from Chapter 2, Victims and Offenders)

RISK FACTORS

VICTIM CHARACTERISTICS
See also Chapter 2, Victims and Offenders.

— Most trafficking victims are women and children.

— Most come from less economically advanced countries or countries characterized by social chaos.

— Some, such as Native American girls and Canadian women, are citizens or permanent residents of more economically advanced countries.

— Special at-risk groups:

1. Children who self-identify as gay

2. Those who cross international borders in pursuit of alcohol, drugs, or sex

3. Foreign children brought into the United States legally who join the ranks of street children because their visa has expired

ENVIRONMENTAL INFLUENCES
Nigeria

— Nigerian women are lured to Europe with promises of higher earnings working in factories, offices, farms, and as dancers or entertainers in nightclubs.

— Once in Europe, the women are sold into sexual slavery to pay off immigration costs (Aghatise, 2004).

— Nigerian women may be forced to swear during black magic juju rites not to reveal who trafficked them or for which madam they work.

Mexico

— Mexico is an origin and a destination for victims of human trafficking.

1. Mexico is used as a transit country for victims from Asia and Eastern Europe on the way to the United States or Canada (Estes, 2005; USDOS, 2004).

2. Belize, El Salvador, Guatemala, and Honduras are the primary countries of origin for trafficked persons.

3. Victims enter through Tapachula, Chiapas, and other southern border communities.

— Most children who engage in survival sex and other sex-for-money exchanges do so because of familial poverty (Azaola, 2001, 2003a,b; Azaola & Estes, 2003).

— Pervasiveness of drug use among street youths is a central component of exploitation of children in Mexico. Children addicted to drugs before exploitation often are prostituted to make enough money to support their addictions (Azaola, 2003a,b; Negrete, 2001).

— The private travel and tourism industry plays a key role in Mexico's challenges with CSE. Ninety-three percent of CSE activities take place in hotels, with employees and managers ignoring the situation. Exploited children may live and work in the same hotel (Azaola, 2001).

— Pedophiles and preferential child sex abusers often come to Mexico as tourists so they can have sex with children (Azaola, 2003b).

1. Although not authorized to provide sexual services, massage parlors, escort services, and modeling agencies promote sex with children and do so openly in the media (Comisión de Derechos Humanos del Distrito Federal, 1996).

2. Sex tourists, most of whom are male, often are richer than the children they exploit and take advantage of destitute, abandoned, and neglected children.

United States and Canada

— Most people trafficked into Canada for sexual purposes come from China, Thailand, Cambodia, the Philippines, Russia, Korea, and Eastern Europe, and the majority are moved into the United States (US DOS, 2003).

— Sexual trafficking of children is especially serious in Canada's larger cities.

— A few children from the United States are abducted and taken into Canada.

— The role of nonfinancial factors is especially important for understanding the sexual exploitation of children from middle-income and upper-income households in the United States and Canada.

— The USDOS classifies countries of origin and destination into a 3-tier system that reflects each country's degree of compliance with basic laws of United States regarding trafficking and treatment of trafficking victims.

1. 140 countries with a minimum of 100 confirmed internal cases of trafficking with a United States nexus are included (**Table 6-1**).

2. The system is still in the initial stages of development but is highly effective as a diplomatic tool for the State Department working with other governments to decrease trafficking (Bishop, 2003).

3. The United States spends more than $70 million annually to halt influx of trafficking victims from other countries (USDOS, 2004). Most of that money is awarded to private organizations that serve trafficking victims directly.

— First responders (medical personnel, social workers, law enforcement officers, ministers, good Samaritans) have an increased exposure to opportunities to identify victims (**Table 6-2**).

PROCESS
— Common characteristics shared by trafficking victims:

1. Are illiterate, unable to speak English, and come from impoverished and desperate circumstances

Table 6-1. 3-Tier Classification System

Tier 1	Countries that fully comply with the Trafficking Victims Protection Act's (TVPA's) minimum standards for the elimination of trafficking.
Tier 2	Countries that do not fully comply with the TVPA's minimum standards but are making efforts to bring themselves into compliance.
Tier 2 (Watch List)	Countries on Tier 2 requiring special scrutiny because of the high or increasing number of victims; failure to provide evidence of increasing efforts to combat trafficking in persons; or an assessment as Tier 2 based on commitments to take action over the next year.
Tier 3	Countries that neither satisfy the minimum standards nor demonstrate a significant effort to come into compliance; countries are subject to potential nonhumanitarian and nontrade sanctions.

Data from USDOS, 2004.

2. Are children, because they are helpless and suggestible

3. Work long hours for little or no salary

4. Are fearful of employers

5. Are restricted in movement and/or being watched or guarded by other employees or family members

6. Appear haggard or fatigued, or display bruising or other evidence of injury

7. Are withdrawn and afraid of contact with unsanctioned outsiders

8. Have statements and attempts at communication stifled or censored by others (deBaca & Tisi, 2002; Venkatraman, 2003)

— Human trafficking operations and their victims remain largely underground.

1. They are often concealed from sight in places such as private homes and back rooms of seemingly legitimate businesses.

Table 6-2. Contexts in Which Child Victims of Trafficking Are Encountered

In a study aimed at identifying juvenile trafficking victims, the United States Conference of Catholic Bishops and the Institute for the Study of International Migration (ISIM) at Georgetown University identified 16 contexts in which law enforcement and social service agencies could encounter child victims of trafficking. The identified locations and groups include the following:

1. Hospital emergency rooms
2. Child protective services agencies
3. State and local juvenile justice departments
4. Domestic violence centers
5. Covenant House type shelters
6. Ethnic community-based organizations
7. Churches and religious centers
8. Healthcare providers
9. School counselor offices
10. Refugee service providers
11. Labor unions/garment industry workers
12. Legal aid agencies
13. Street outreach programs
14. Soup kitchens/homeless shelters
15. Domestic servants
16. Prostituted adults

Data from Bump & Duncan, 2003.

2. Victims may be overseen by guards who monitor their movements and contacts.

3. These factors plus fear of law enforcement officials and/or retaliation by traffickers contribute to invisibility of victims.

— Trafficking offenses masquerade as other crimes.

1. These include vice crimes, domestic violence, immigration offenses, and other types of criminal activity.

2. Investigators and prosecutors may encounter situations when a victim's neighbor calls the police to respond to a domestic violence offense.

— Certain facts, such as a significant salary, failure to flee the trafficking situation despite multiple opportunities, and initial consent to substandard working conditions or commercial sex, do not necessarily undercut the viability of a trafficking prosecution. If unlawful means are used to overcome the victim's will and force performance, statutory requirements for slavery and trafficking offenses can be met.

— Crimes must be accurately identified so victims can receive specialized assistance.

1. Trafficking victims are considered victims of violent crime and are handled separately from victims and witnesses in immigration and other cases.

2. Victims are often brainwashed into believing law enforcement officials will behave punitively.

3. Before the Trafficking Victims Protecton Act (TVPA), some victims were placed in immigration detention while the authorities attempted to find suitable housing and financial assistance to meet their needs.

4. Victims would sometimes lie or attempt to mislead investigators, risking exposure to criminal liability and/or administrative actions by immigration courts.

5. The TVPA confers special victim status so qualified individuals are streamlined through government channels to receive immigration benefits, psychological counseling, employment authorization and training, housing and food assistance, medical care, and other benefits.

6. This special status is not tied to successful prosecution of a case; victims access temporary immigration, healthcare, employment and other benefits even while the investigation is pending.

— Federal law enforcement authorities have noted a pattern of recurrence in certain industries or services such as massage parlors, strip clubs, brothels, garment manufacturing plants (sweatshops), farms and other agribusinesses that employ migrant labor, restaurants that employ busboys and dishwashers, and homes that employ domestic help.

— Some apparently benign businesses may offer commercial sexual services (deBaca & Tisi, 2002).

— As a result of the Jacob Wetterling Act and Megan's Law, some offenders leave the United States to have sex with children. The rationalization is that it will be easier to have sex with children in third tier countries that do not have proactive or reactive laws forbidding the prostitution of children and youths than in those that have strict laws.

INVESTIGATION

— Formal questioning of suspected victims is best left to investigators. Threshold questions may include (deBaca & Tisi, 2002; Venkatraman, 2003):

1. How did you come to work for [the defendant]?

2. Describe your work.

3. Were you paid?

4. Could you come and go at will?

5. Could you talk to anyone you wanted to talk to?

6. How did you arrive in the United States?

7. Did anyone take your passport or papers?

— If victims resist answering, appear to be withholding information, or are not being truthful:

1. Reassure them that they are not in trouble.

2. Do not persist in questioning them.

— All cases warrant immediate contact with law enforcement officials, and any basic questions should be asked through a trustworthy interpreter.

— Law enforcement officers involved in vice operations or other professionals who work on vice-related issues should note particularly young-looking prostituted individuals even if they claim to be adults.

— Sexual abuse of trafficking victims even in cases not involving sex trafficking and/or commercial sex has been noted by US Department of Justice (USDOJ) attorneys in several recent matters, particularly cases involving juvenile domestic servants.

1. Such workers are arguably the most cloistered and isolated of all victimized groups, as they normally work in private homes.

2. These victims may be visible when working in the yard, walking a dog, taking children to school, or tending children in public places (malls, parks).

3. Be aware of domestic workers, especially juveniles who may be introduced to visitors or other inquiring parties as relatives.

4. Traffickers often procure their kin for trafficking into domestic servitude, other labor, or commercial sex (Dhakal, 2004). A claim of kinship can be a ruse to mislead inquiring individuals or the reason a victim was targeted to work for the trafficker in the first place.

LEGAL STATUS
See **Table 6-3**.

INTERPOL

— Takes on the role of educator and facilitator of crime investigations.

— Is the international source of the most comprehensive array of information about child sexual exploitation, especially crimes against children, trafficking of women, and human smuggling.

— Provides missing children posters to help investigators identify victims (**Table 6-4**).

Table 6-3. Comparison of Legal Approaches to Trafficking in the United States, Canada, and Mexico

UNITED STATES

— Recently established program offices:

1. *Office to Monitor and Combat Trafficking in Persons of the USDOS.* Leads American antitrafficking efforts and assists President's Interagency Task Force to Monitor and Combat Trafficking in Persons, which is responsible for monitoring and combating trafficking.

2. *Trafficking in Persons Report Section of the USDOS.* Collects data and corresponds with governments to assess progress in combating trafficking; issues annual report noting compliance with TVPA requirements.

3. *International Programs Section of USDOS.* Promotes and coordinates US antitrafficking efforts.

4. *Public Diplomacy and Outreach Section of USDOS.* Develops public-private partnerships with American and international nongovernmental organizations working to eliminate international trafficking of people.

5. *Specialized antitrafficking units part of USDOJ, US Department of Homeland Security, US Department of Health and Human Services (USDHHS), US Agency for International Development, and US Department of Labor.*

6. *Prosecutorial Remedies and Other Tools to end the Exploitation of Children Today (PROTECT) Act of 2003.* Expands AMBER Alert system nationally; makes it a crime for citizens or legal residents of United States to engage in sexual acts with a child younger than 18 years in a foreign country; removes legal requirements related to proof of intention to engage in such acts before travel; strengthens sentencing guideline provisions for offenders; adds "two strikes and you're out" provision for repeat offenders of sex crimes against children plus mandatory sentencing requirements; provides law enforcement authorities with new tools to deal with trafficking of children for sexual purposes.

(continued)

Table 6-3. *(continued)*

UNITED STATES

— Number of cases of juvenile prostitution, child trafficking, and child sex tourism prosecuted under federal laws relatively low; numerous cases of electronic child pornography prosecuted.

— Those certified as victims by the USDHHS are entitled to services and benefits due refugees other than the Reception and Placement Program. Certification is required for receiving a T-visa, which permits trafficking victims to remain in the United States.

CANADA

— Immigration & Refugee Protection Act (IRPA) of 2002 references best interests of child, expands definition of dependent children, and clarifies provisions related to international adoptions where children could be at risk for exploitation.

— Recent laws were expanded to prohibit aiding, abetting, counseling, compelling, or luring those younger than 18 years into prostitution. Penalties especially severe when force, coercion, or threats are used to compel children to engage in prostitution, pornography, and sexual trafficking. Prohibits Canadian citizens and permanent residents from participating in international sexual tourism.

MEXICO

— Laws prohibiting international trafficking in people poorly enforced. Usually involve deportation back to Mexico of people who illegally enter the United States or Canada.

— Federal penal code covers procuring, facilitating, or forcing a child younger than 18 years to perform acts related to pornography, prostitution, or consumption of narcotics or to commit criminal acts. Punishments of at least 5 years in prison.

— Trafficking in children not considered a crime in all 31 Mexican states. Children older than 16 years not protected under most of Mexico's laws.

— Mexican legal system prosecutes few child sexual exploiters and brings to trial even fewer. Children who press charges are often threatened by exploiters and drop the cases.

Table 6-4. Interpol's Tools for Protecting Children

Tool	Description
Individual notices	Provide specific information about a person who has committed a crime, is missing, or whose body cannot be identified; includes identity, physical description, photograph and fingerprints if available. Types of notices are wanted (red), enquiry (blue), warning (green), missing persons (yellow), and unidentified body (black). Also periodic newsletter for law enforcement officials with information about current crime trends, international yellow notices, and Interpol posters.
International yellow notices and Interpol poster on missing children	Circulated to police departments that handle disappearances and those in border regions. 12 photographs of children missing for 5 years or more; some age-progressed. Intended to be circulated to general public, displayed in railway stations and airports, published in newspapers, or distributed to nongovernmental organizations that help search for missing persons.
International green notices	Provide information about offenders likely to commit more crimes. Person concerned has convictions for offenses committed in at least 3 different countries or has been revealed in an inquiry during an investigation or court case regarding someone else or has proved links with organized crime. Apply to perpetrators of crimes against children. Serve as working tool for combating sexual abuse of children by individuals who operate in more than one country.
Computer systems	Provide technical and professional assistance to member nations. Implement automated search facility. Give rapid access to information.

(continued)

Table 6-4. *(continued)*	

TOOL	DESCRIPTION
Data entry, electronic archiving, and automatic consultation	Maintain a computer record of names and aliases of people implicated in international cases; record of offenses classified by type of offense, place of commission, and modus operandi; record of identification numbers noted in course of police investigations; file that contains prints of all 10 fingers of various international offenders; photograph file for specialized and habitual offenders as well as missing persons; system of electronic archiving with computerized indexing; electronic text and image server for instant and remote consultation of a database of selected information.

— Maintains Web site of legislation data and commonly used trafficking routes for smuggling of people, drugs, and other contraband.

1. Though routes are carefully defined, when people are preparing to reach Western countries, land travel is forfeited for the more expensive but successful air travel.

2. Interpol notes that trafficking networks are focusing more on Central and South America, where they can maintain links to Mexico and North America.

— Uses the definitions for human trafficking included in the United Nations Convention Against Transnational Organized Crime, which distinguish between smuggling of migrants and trafficking of people.

1. Smuggling of migrants:

   A. Procurement, for financial or material benefit, of illegal entry of a person into a region where the person is not a national or permanent resident (Children and human trafficking, 2004)

   B. Increasingly sophisticated, moving more people daily, and receiving higher profits

C. Reflects migration from least developed countries of Asia, Africa, South America, and Eastern Europe to Western Europe, Australia, and North America

D. Often involves inhuman conditions, such as transport via overcrowded trucks or boats, and subsequent deaths

E. Migrants arriving at destination country are illegal immigrants, completely dependent on the smugglers

F. Migrants often become indentured servants for years to pay off debts

G. Family members in home countries sometimes threatened and forced to pay to save smuggled relative's life

2. Trafficking of persons is the "recruitment, transportation, transfer, harboring or receipt of persons, by means of the threat or use of force (or other forms of coercion or abduction), fraud, deception, the abuse of power or of a position of vulnerability, or the giving or receiving of payments or benefits to achieve the consent of a person having control over another person for the purpose of exploitation," including at least prostitution or other forms of sexual exploitation, forced labor, slavery or similar practices, servitude, or the removal of organs (Protocol to Prevent, 2000).

— Barriers to international cooperation:

1. Varying structures of national law enforcement agencies so the authority of various departments is unclear

2. Different languages

3. Varied legal systems and ages of consent

— Interpol continues to lobby politically for stronger international legislation on human trafficking. Consistent arrests and prosecutions are a goal of the international community through the structure provided on a global basis by Interpol and other policing and advocacy agencies.

LEGAL RESULTS FOR OFFENDERS
— They are punished more stringently than immigration violators or domestic batterers.

— Most offenses carry a maximum statutory penalty of 20 years imprisonment; some juvenile sex trafficking has a maximum term of life imprisonment.

— The TVPA requires defendants convicted of trafficking crimes to pay mandatory restitution to their victims.

LEGAL RESULTS FOR VICTIMS
— Many victims whose cases are resolved have options they never had before, making them less vulnerable to revictimization.

Table 6-5. Other Assistance Available to Trafficking Victims

T-visa benefits impose the additional requirement of establishing extreme hardship upon removal to the victim's home country. Not all victims have chosen to remain in the United States; some have requested repatriation to their home countries during the investigation or after its conclusion. In one case, a group of juvenile victims requested to be reunited with their families in their native country though the victims expressed a willingness to return to the United States to testify against the traffickers. In another investigation, a victim of Indo-Nepalese origin requested repatriation to India so she could be reunited with her daughter. In such instances, federal personnel have assisted in securing victim benefits pending repatriation.

Despite the requirements for continued presence and T-visa status, victims can access immediate services upon liberation even before receiving official "certification" as a victim of a severe form of trafficking. The USDOJ has funded grants for emergency medical attention, food, shelter, vocational and language training, mental health counseling, and legal support available during the precertification stage. The Office of Victims of Crime provides grants to nongovernmental agencies for the specific purpose of assisting victims "between the period of time they are encountered by law enforcement, and when they are 'certified' to receive other benefits through the Department of Health and Human Services" (Trafficking in persons, 2004).

— Different forms of relief, which involve separate and distinct requirements, are available to victims.

1. Generally, the TVPA requires that a victim must be defined as a "victim of a severe form of trafficking" who is a potential witness in a case (to qualify for temporary immigration benefits under the "continued presence" immigration provision) and/or one who demonstrates a willingness to assist law enforcement officials in their investigation and prosecution efforts (to qualify for longer-term and potentially permanent T-visa benefits) (**Table 6-5**).

2. Any law enforcement official encountering a potential trafficking situation must determine whether the situation involves a "victim of a severe form of trafficking," which means the victim was subjected to the following offenses (22 USC § 7102 [2004]):

    A. A commercial sex act induced by force, fraud, or coercion, or one in which the person induced to perform such an act is younger than 18 years

    B. The recruitment, harboring, transportation, provision, or obtaining of a person for labor or services, through the use of force, fraud, or coercion for the purpose of subjection to involuntary servitude, peonage, debt bondage, or slavery

— The law enforcement agency then works with the USDHHS to certify the victim to receive state refugee benefits in the locality where the victim resides.

— Violations that qualify for classification as trafficking crimes, which are not mutually exclusive, entitling victims to receive benefits, include:

1. *Involuntary servitude.* A victim is required to work or perform services through force, threats of force, or threats of legal coercion (18 USC § 1584).

2. *Forced labor.* A victim is required to work under threats of "serious harm," including psychologically coercive ploys aimed at a victim's family members, and/or schemes, plans, or patterns

intended to lead a victim to believe that the victim or another person would suffer serious harm or physical restraint for failing to perform the requested services (18 USC § 1589).

3. *Sex trafficking of children by force, fraud, or coercion.* A victim is required to perform a commercial sex act through force, fraud, or coercion, or a minor victim is required to perform a commercial sex act (18 USC § 1591).

— With juvenile trafficking victims, separate benefits apply.

1. Minor victims can participate in the Unaccompanied Refugee Minor Program run by the USDHHS. They do not require certification to receive these benefits.

2. The process is even more streamlined for children so they can access the needed benefits quickly. Victims aged 16 to 24 years who have work permits may be eligible for Job Corps, a program run by the US Department of Labor.

HOW TO OBTAIN HELP

STEPS TO TAKE

— Alert law enforcement officials.

— In an emergency when the victim must be liberated immediately, call emergency services.

— The case can be initiated through the USDOJ Trafficking in Persons and Worker Exploitation Complaint Line (888-428-7581).

1. Operates 24 hours and is staffed during business hours by Civil Rights Division

2. Uses TTY services for the hearing impaired and offers 150 languages

3. Accesses services of prosecutors who work exclusively on human trafficking prosecutions plus full-time Victim Witness Specialist to assist in obtaining benefits, accessing representation, finding helpful social service groups near residence, and arranging for competent and neutral interpretation services

4. All complaints confidential

— Federal investigations can be initiated by notifying field offices of various federal law enforcement agencies.

END CHILD PROSTITUTION, CHILD PORNOGRAPHY AND TRAFFICKING OF CHILDREN FOR SEXUAL PURPOSES (ECPAT) CAMPAIGN

— Goals:

1. To raise international awareness of problem

2. To build active grassroots advocacy groups

3. To effect a global network

4. To encourage governmental organizations (GOs) and communities to implement laws and policies to stop child sexual exploitation

— Has facilitated the formation of national grassroots ECPAT campaigns worldwide:

1. All shaped by social, cultural, political context but share vision

2. Aim to educate and lobby locally within their own countries and to support international actions to pressure world leaders and GOs to eradicate child sex tourism

— Takes a multidisciplinary approach:

1. Work with community groups, government officials, individuals in the private sector, and people in media industry

2. Use mass media channels and partner with world media organizations to expose the involvement of each country's nationals in child sex tourism and convince GOs to take proactive investigative and prosecution measures

— Formed a working relationship with the tourism industry and now addresses sexual exploitation of children in that industry.

1. Well received by key international travel and tourism industry groups

2. Educate tourism professionals about and take action to prevent sexual abuse of children in tourism

3. Distribute printed materials via travel agents, in airports, through visa and passport offices, and at other travel exit points

— Created Internet platform offering information about sexual exploitation of children to educate public and guide actions against CSE.

— Actions have led to a significant number of prosecutions under child sex tourism laws in sending countries.

— For destination countries:

1. Seeks to deter and identify child sex tourists

2. Promotes the enactment and enforcement of child protection legislation

3. Supported by GOs that send out strong messages to child sex tourists

— Other sex tourism incentives:

1. *Child Wise Tourism Program.* Training and network development program that seeks to build partnerships among government and nongovernment agencies and the tourism industry to protect children from sexual abuse. Focuses on training people who work on tourism's front line (hotel staff members, tourism managers, tourist police officers, tourism trainers, trainers in tourism institutions, others in industry).

2. *Association of Southeast Asian Nations (ASEAN) Regional Think Tank.* Provides organized venues for communication among government national tourism authorities, travel industry representatives, and child protection agency officials for the purpose of developing and strengthening working relationships and stressing the reality of a need to prevent child sex tourism.

3. *Association of Southeast Asian Nations (ASEAN) Travellers Code.* Promoted to encourage prevention of abuse and exploitation of people, promotion of human rights (especially those of women and children), and consideration of activities they undertake and the businesses they support while traveling.

4. *Stop It Now.* Provides the first helpline for individuals and communities attempting to accept responsibility for the sexual abuse of children. This international organization provides information on all aspects of sexual abuse and sexual exploitation, facilitates mental health contact information, and explains the legal system for those who are attempting to cease offending behaviors.

REFERENCES

Aghatise E. Trafficking for prostitution in Italy: possible effects of government proposals for legalization of brothels. *Violence Against Women.* 2004;10:1126-1155.

Azaola E. La explotación sexual commercial de niños en México: situación general de la infancia. In: Azaola E, Estes RJ, eds. *La Infancia Como Mercancia Sexual. México, Canadá, Estados Unidos.* Mexico City, Mexico: Siglo Veintiuno Editores; 2003a:140-155.

Azaola E. La explotación sexual de niños en las fronteras. In: Azaola E, Estes RJ, eds. *La Infancia Como Mercancia Sexual. México, Canadá, Estados Unidos.* Mexico City, Mexico: Siglo Veintiuno Editores; 2003b:240-322.

Azaola E. *Stolen Childhood: Girl and Boy Victims of Sexual Exploitation in Mexico.* Mexico City, Mexico: United Nations Children's Fund (UNICEF); 2001.

Azaola E, Estes RJ, eds. *La Infancia Como Mercancia Sexual. México, Canadá, Estados Unidos.* Mexico City, Mexico: Siglo Veintiuno Editores; 2003.

Bishop C. The Trafficking Victims Protection Act of 2000: three years later. *Int Migration.* 2003;41(6):219-231.

Bump M, Duncan J. Conference on identifying and serving child victims of trafficking. *Int Migr* [serial online]. December 2003;41:201-218. Available at: http://www.blackwell-synergy.com/links/doi/10.1111/j.0020-7985.2003.00266.x/enhancedabs/. Accessed August 9, 2004.

Children and human trafficking. Interpol Web site. Available at: http://www.Interpol.int/Public/THB/default.asp. Accessed December 31, 2004.

Comisión de Derechos Humanos del Distrito Federal. *Al Otro Lado de la Calle: Prostitución de Menroes en La Merced*. Mexico City, Mexico: Comisión de Derechos Humanos del Distrito Federal-UNICEF; 1996.

deBaca L, Tisi A. Working together to stop modern-day slavery. *Police Chief Magazine*. August 2002;69(8):79-80.

Dhakal S. Nepal's victims of trafficking shy away from justice. *One World South Asia*. January 8, 2004. Available at: http://southasia. oneworld.net/article/view/76359/1/1. Accessed August 9, 2004.

18 USC § 1584 (2000).

18 USC § 1589 (2004).

18 USC § 1589 et seq.

18 USC § 1591 (2004).

Estes RJ. *Social Development in Hong Kong: The Unfinished Agenda*. New York, NY: Oxford University Press; 2005

Graycar A. Trafficking in human beings. Paper presented at: International Conference on Migration, Culture, and Crime; July 7, 1999; Israel.

Lederer L. *Human Rights Report on Trafficking of Women and Children*. Baltimore, Md: Johns Hopkins University, The Paul H. Nitze School of Advanced International Studies; 2001.

Negrete N. *Explotación Sexual Comercial de la Niñez en el sur de México y Centroamérica*. San José, Costa Rica: ECPAT-Casa Alianza; 2001.

Protocol to Prevent, Suppress and Punish Trafficking in Persons, Especially Women and Children, Supplementing the United Nations Convention Against Transnational Organized Crime. December 2000. United Nations Office on Drugs and Crime web-site. Available at:

http://www.unodc.org/pdf/crime/a_res_55/res5525e.pdf. Accessed August 20, 2003.

Raymond JG. Prostitution on demand: legalizing the buyers as sexual consumers. *Violence Against Women.* 2004;10:1156-1186.

Richard AO. International Trafficking in Women to the US: A Contemporary Manifestation of Slavery and Organized Crime. Washington, DC: US State Dept Bureau of Intelligence and Research; 1999.

Schloenhardt A. The business of migration: organized crime and illegal migration in Australia and the Asia-Pacific region. Paper presented at: University of Adelaide Law School; May, 1999; Adelaide, Australia.

Trafficking in persons. Office of Victims of Crime Web site. Available at: http://www.ojp.usdoj.gov/ovc/help/tip.htm#4. Accessed August 9, 2004.

22 USC § 7102 (2004).

US Department of State. *Trafficking in Persons Report, 2003.* Washington, DC: US Dept of State, Office of the Under Secretary for Global Affairs; 2003.

US Department of State. *Trafficking in Persons Report, 2004.* Washington, DC: US Dept of State, Office of the Under Secretary for Global Affairs; 2004.

Venkatraman BA. Human trafficking: a guide to detecting, investigating and punishing modern-day slavery. *Police Chief Magazine.* December 2003;70(12):41.

Yoon Y. *International Sexual Slavery.* Washington, DC: CG Issue Overviews; 1997.

Chapter 7

MEDICAL ISSUES

Sharon W. Cooper, MD, FAAP
Nancy D. Kellogg, MD
Elizabeth J. Letourneau, PhD
David S. Prescott, LICSW
F. Bruce Watkins, MD

PRINCIPLES OF CARE FOR VICTIMS AND SUSPECTED OFFENDERS

— Medical care for children involved in adverse circumstances (runaways, homeless, engaging in survival sex or sex for drugs, having sexually transmitted diseases [STDs], substance abuse, crime, and violence):

1. Care begins with a medical emergency or compulsory examination after incarceration.

2. Risk of medical problems is significantly increased.

3. Most prostituted adolescents consider their health to be excellent or good (Unger et al, 1998). Their lack of concern reflects denial, ignorance, or inability to understand the consequences of their lifestyle.

— Children and adolescents may be reluctant to seek help and unwilling to give information that may result in arrest, placement in a shelter, or a return to their families.

— Suspect assessments are usually focused on proving that the individual did or did not commit a crime.

OBTAINING HISTORY

— Be sensitive to victims' age, race, gender, sexual orientation, national origin, and mental status.

— Ask open-ended questions to reconstruct history (**Tables 7-1** and **7-2**).

— Inform patients that absolute confidentiality is not assured, as history, physical examination, and medical records could become court evidence.

— **Table 7-3** gives tips.

— In the concluding interview:

1. Summarize the proposed diagnosis.

2. Outline the next step (physical examination) and its purpose.

3. Listen to and discuss any questions or concerns that patients may have.

4. Emphasize the importance of compliance.

5. Outline future appointments, follow-up, and counseling.

ASSESSMENT

— All suspected victims of child or adolescent sexual abuse should be evaluated by a pediatrician or mental health provider so treatment and safety needs, especially degree of parental support, can be assessed (American Academy of Pediatrics [AAP] Committee on Child Abuse and Neglect, 1999).

— Clinical management options:

1. Need for forensic evidence collection and the clinician's comfort level dictate whether a clinician refers a child to specialized child abuse evaluation center or elects to conduct all or part of the medical examination.

2. Multidisciplinary teams, which are generally found in hospital settings or at a child advocacy center, may evaluate all child and adolescent victims; referrals may provide the best care for victims of acute and chronic sexual abuse.

— An assessment is intended to gather objective evidence to corroborate and confirm a victim's accusations (**Table 7-4**).

Table 7-1. Obtaining a Victim's History

When interviewing a victim, an alleged perpetrator, or other sources, an investigative team must observe the following indicators and record them in writing and on audiotape or videotape.

AVAILABLE HISTORICAL AND INFORMATIONAL SOURCES

— The victim
— The perpetrator and/or coconspirator
— The authorities (ie, police officer, security officer, teacher)
— A witness or collateral observer
— Family member
— Outreach worker
— Friend and/or companion (ie, confidant)

THE ASSESSMENT TEAM SHOULD OBSERVE AND DOCUMENT ALL SUBTLE CLUES FROM THE SOURCE

— Victim is emotional, afraid, or stoic
— Victim is communicative
— Victim is aggressive and/or confrontational
— Victim is under the influence of drugs or alcohol
— Victim changes details
— Victim has trigger points or issues
— Victim has mood changes
— Victim is incensed
— Victim is unclear, illogical, or incoherent
— Victim seems abrupt or hurried
— Victim seems to be protecting someone
— Victim has an inappropriate affect
— Victim is clutching something physical
— Victim is avoiding a particular subject

— Role of the examiner does not include judging, exhibiting a negative attitude, lecturing, admonishing the patient, or using leading questions and statements.

— An examiner must be an independent observer, sensitive, gentle, communicative, problem-oriented, suspicious, intuitive, and open-minded.

Table 7-2. Revealing Questions That May Provide Further Information About Abuse

Interviewers should avoid questions that require one-word answers. If "yes" or "no" is all the patient provides, question futher to get more in-depth answers.

HOME ENVIRONMENT

— Where do you live?
— How long have you lived there?
— With whom do you live?
— Describe your relationships with parents and siblings.
— What are your responsibilities in the home?
— Do you receive an allowance?
— Describe your daily schedule.
— Have you run away from home?

EDUCATION

— Do you attend school?
— Describe your behavior at school.
— Describe your grades.
— What subjects do you find interesting?
— What subjects do you find boring?
— Have you ever been suspended from school?
— Are you involved in any after-school activities?
— Do you have a job?
— Are you involved in sports?
— Do you plan to pursue more or advanced schooling?

ACTIVITIES

— What do you like to do for fun?
— Are you involved in out-of-school sports or teams?
— Are you involved in any organizations (eg, scouts, church, community, gangs)?
— Do you like to read? If yes, what do you like to read?
— What type of music do you prefer?
— Do you have a car available to you? If yes, who owns the car?
— Do you have any hobbies?
— Describe your friends (eg, Who are they? What do your friends do?).
— Who is your best friend?
— How much time do you spend with friends?   *(continued)*

Table 7-2. *(continued)*

— How much time do you spend watching television?
— What do you like to watch on television?
— How much time do you spend playing video games?
— What type of video games do you like to play?
— Do you have an income? If yes, what is the source of this income?
— Are you a member of any groups?

DRUGS

— Do your peers use drugs? If yes, what type of drugs do they use?
— Do members of your family use drugs? If yes, what types of drugs do they use?
— Do you or have you used drugs? If yes, what type of drugs do you use and when do you use them? How do you pay for these drugs?

SEX

— Do you date?
— Have you had previous sexual experiences? If yes, what type of experience have you had? How many sexual partners have you had altogether? When was your first sexual experience?
— Are any of your friends sexually active? If yes, what type of sexual experiences do they have?
— Are you currently sexually involved with someone?
— What is your sexual preference?
— Have you ever had a sexually transmitted disease? If yes, what type have you had?
— Do you use contraception? If yes, what type do you use?
— How frequently do you have sexual intercourse?
— Have you ever been pregnant?
— Have you ever had an abortion?
— What are your feelings about intercourse?

SUICIDE

— Do you currently have any suicidal ideas or thoughts?
— Have you ever tried to commit suicide?
— Have you ever planned a suicide attempt?
— Would you ever kill yourself?
— Have any of your friends ever attempted to commit suicide or succeeded in commiting suicide?

Table 7-3. Interviewer Tips for Obtaining a History

— Establish rapport with the patient; share common ground.
— Refer the patient to someone else if the situation is uncomfortable for either participant.
— Ask with whom the patient would feel most comfortable or prefer to have ask these questions.
— Select the first setting for the interview in a nonmedical environment and then move to a medical space for the physical examination.
— The interview should be conducted in a one-on-one setting.
— A repeated interview with a chaperone may provide additional information.
— If the child is mature enough and communicative, consider using the HEADSS (**H**ome, **E**ducation/employment, **A**ctivity, **D**rugs, **S**exuality, **S**uicide/depression screen) interview line of questioning for the personal history.
— Remember that the personal history provides a context for the recollection of events.
— Summarize and restate the objectives and goals of the interview and physical examination recurrently.
— Determine the immediacy of the physical examination according to the amount of time that has elapsed since an event.
— Always keep the objectives and goals in mind in selecting questions and doing tests.
— Assure confidentiality; however, explain what information cannot be kept confidential.
— Avoid interruptions to maintain rapport.
— Take notes regarding observations; develop a timeline of events.
— Mention previous history issues.
— Avoid the role of the surrogate parent or that of a pal or friend.
— Act as an advocate.
— Circumvent power struggles.
— Listen without interruption.
— Ask open-ended questions.

(continued)

Table 7-3. *(continued)*

— Ask whether the patient is in danger; this directs the thrust of the investigation.
— Inform the patient that some personal but important questions will be asked.

Data from Adams, 2001; American Academy of Pediatrics, Committee on Child Abuse and Neglect, 1999; Neinstein & Ratner Kaufman, 2002; Patel & Minshall, 2001.

Table 7-4. A Physical Examiner's Checklist

When performing a physical examination on a child victim of sexual assault, the physical examiner should:

— Recruit the patient for compliance.
— Describe the trauma sites.
— Describe the degree of injury.
— Describe the pattern of injury.
— Propose the mechanism of injury.
— Observe whether the injury is acute or nonacute.
— Decide whether the child is in danger.
— Always be aware of the chain of evidence.

Additionally, the physical examiner should remember the following facts:

— Many child molestations are nonviolent and do not involve visible genital injury.
— From the child's point of view, the physical examination should not be worse than the molestation.
— Being very careful, gentle, and sensitive is important.
— When genital injury is apparent, an age-appropriate differential diagnosis should be generated.
— The motive for evidence collection, taking a history, and conducting a physical examination may change with time.

— Promote child and family compliance by acting as victims' advocate.

— Allow the presence of a chaperone and/or assistant during procedure.

Table 7-5. Objectives for Conducting a Physical Examination on an Assault Victim

— Diagnose and treat the physical, emotional, and behavioral consequences of abuse.

— Confirm and validate statements made in the interview.

— Establish the basic condition of the victim and recognize any underlying health problems.

— Acquire and preserve forensic evidence.

— Establish present baseline status in reference to sexually transmitted diseases, pregnancy, body systems and their functions, since many tests require serial observations.

— Plan prophylaxis and/or preemptive therapy.

— Assess the amount of objective corroborating evidence.

— Why examine: See **Table 7-5**.

— Initial decisions regarding examination procedure:

1. *Where to examine.* Consider the relevant history, time elapsed since alleged assault, patient's age, availability of evidence, and psychological state of victim. Patients place a high value on convenience and comfort after an alleged assault (Heger & Emans, 1992).

2. *When to examine.* The earlier it takes place, the more likely evidence will be recovered and the findings will be useful in diagnosis or litigation. Sexual assaults often have no anogenital findings, but immediate interview and physical examination of untouched clothing and debris may offer clues. Conduct the examination before victims clean up and bathe.

3. *How to examine.* Check vital signs, observe, and document physical findings from head to toe. Remain observant and carefully collect all physical evidence. Perform the genital examination last (Lenahan et al, 1998).

— An examiner must also decide:

1. Whether to use a speculum.

2. Whether to obtain samples for culture and wet mount from the vagina.

3. Whether and how to collect samples of specimens found on victims; samples can be analyzed to identify DNA component.

4. Whether to use Wood's light to reveal otherwise invisible dried bodily secretions on victims so samples can be obtained, preserved, and perhaps used to identify the perpetrator.

5. Whether to test and how to conduct and follow up on a test, since many cultures and serum assays require serial studies to verify transmission, encouraging a repeat examination.

    A. Initial tests may assess immediate or baseline status.

    B. Appropriate tests/cultures should be chosen and omitted according to clinical circumstances.

CLINICAL APPROACH

— Position patient on chaperone's lap with knees spread apart (frog-leg) to increase comfort and convenience.

— Use the TEAMSTAT approach (**Table 7-6**).

— Assess for drug or alcohol use (**Tables** 7-7 and **7-8**).

Assessing for Nongenital Injuries

— Swab suspicious areas during forensic evidence collection and submit to test for assailant's saliva (AAP & C Henry Kempe National Center on Child Abuse and Neglect, 1994).

— Types and mechanisms of injuries seen in sexual assault victims are summarized in **Table 7-9**.

— When possible, have an experienced photographer document injuries with 35-mm or digital camera.

1. Label photographs clearly with patient identifier and date.

2. Place ruler/color guide next to each injury.

Table 7-6. The "TEAMSTAT" Approach

Tell them your agenda

Express concern

Assure normalcy of feelings

Medical issues

— Sexual/physical victimization

— Drug and alcohol use

— Psychiatric symptoms and diagnoses

Safety issues

— Family history, support

— Runaway tendencies

Test and treat presumptively

— Sexually transmitted diseases (STDs)

— Pregnancy prophylaxis, birth control

Access appropriate psychological and legal assistance

— Psychiatric assessment

— Reporting requirements

Timely follow-up

— Injuries

— STDs

— Birth control

— Drug and alcohol use

Adapted from Kellogg & Sugarek, 1998.

3. Fully document color, location, and size of injuries on body map.

4. Be aware some deep bruises do not become apparent for 2 to 3 days; document areas of tenderness and follow up with photographs as bruises appear.

5. Avoid precise dating of bruises; they can be described as acute (within 3 days), characterized by edema, violaceous or red-blue

Table 7-7. Symptoms of Drug Use and Withdrawal

SUBSTANCE	INTOXICATION EFFECTS	WITHDRAWAL EFFECTS
Ethanol	— Varies from impaired coordination to stupor — Nausea/vomiting — Hypoglycemia — Gastritis	— Varies; includes headache, tremors, tachycardia, insomnia (delirium tremens is rare)
Marijuana	— Varies from euphoria to paranoia/psychosis — Decreased problem-solving, memory — Increased appetite — Impaired coordination	— Sleep disturbances, tremors, anorexia — Chronic use: decreased motivation, global cognitive impairment, mild feminization, decreased sperm count
Heroin and other opiates	— Respiratory depression/arrest — Pupillary miosis — Impaired mentation — Seizures — Hypotension, brady-cardia, arrhythmias — Chronic use: generalized pruritus, constipation, bronchospasm	— Myalgias — Irritability — Nausea/vomiting — Tremors — Hypertension, tachycardia
Cocaine	— Hyperalertness, euphoria — Insomnia, paranoia, psychosis — Pupillary miosis — Hypertension, tachycardia — Elevated temperature — Coronary vasospasm — Rhabdomyolysis	— Depression, irritability — Tremor — Lethargy — Nausea — Chronic use: unsatisfiable craving for more
Hallucinogens (LSD, PCP)	— Altered visual/auditory sense — Altered mood, sense of time/space	— No specific withdrawal symptoms

(continued)

Table 7-7. *(continued)*

	— Aggressive state (PCP) — Elevated temperature — Tachycardia	
Amphetamines	— Hyperactivity — Irritability, anxiety, panic — Elevated temperature — Hypertension, tachycardia — Insomnia — Anorexia — Seizures, arrhythmias	— Lethargy — Depression — Sweats — Abdominal cramps — Muscle cramps — Hypotension
Depressants (prescription drugs, including sedatives, hypnotics, tranquilizers)	— Similar to ethanol intoxication — Sedation — Ataxia, slurred speech — Respiratory depression	— Similar to ethanol withdrawal — Irritability, tremors, elevated temperature, tachycardia, hypertension — Chronic use: cognitive deficits, motor slowing, incoordination, mood lability
Inhalants (toluene, paint thinner, glue, spray paint, gasoline, freon, propane)	— Euphoria — Hallucinations — Nystagmus — Rhinorrhea — Respiratory depression/arrest	— No specific withdrawal symptoms — Chronic use: tremor, ataxia, peripheral neuropathy, hyperactivity, expressive/receptive processing difficulties, dementia
Other club drugs (Ecstasy, gammahydroxy-butyrate [GHB], ketamine, Rohypnol)	— Tachycardia — Hypertension — Hyperthermia — Confusion/anxiety/paranoia — Heart/kidney failure — Respiratory depression — Amnesia	— No specific withdrawal symptoms

Data from Fishman et al, 1997; Schwartz & Alderman, 1997.

Table 7-8. CRAFFT Screening Test for Adolescent Substance Abuse

C Have you ever ridden in a CAR driven by someone (including yourself) who was "high" or had been using alcohol or drugs?

R Do you ever use alcohol or drugs to RELAX, feel better about yourself, or fit in?

A Do you ever use alcohol/drugs while you are by yourself, ALONE?

F Do you ever FORGET things you did while using alcohol or drugs?

F Do your family or FRIENDS ever tell you that you should cut down on your drinking or drug use?

T Have you gotten into TROUBLE while you were using alcohol or drugs?

Reprinted from CeASAR: The Center for Adolescent Substance Abuse Research, 2003. © Children's Hospital Boston, 2001. Reproduced with permission from the Center for Adolescent Substance Abuse Research, CeASAR, Children's Hospital Boston. For more information, contact info@CRAFFT.org, or visit www.crafft.org.

---

color, and less distinct margins (AAP & C Henry Kempe National Center on Child Abuse and Neglect, 1994).

6. Recent or healed bite marks should be referred to a forensic odontologist for photography and forensic analysis if possible.

Assessing for Genital and Anal Injuries
— Preparing a child for the examination:

1. Show the victim the examination room and any equipment before the medical examination. Include hands-on experience when possible.

2. Prepare the child in the presence of a parent or support person to reduce anxiety.

3. Sedation is usually not needed if a child is properly prepared.

— Positions:

1. *Supine frog-leg position.* Used for smaller prepubertal girls. Child places soles of feet together with knees flexed laterally. Provides an

Table 7-9. Nongenital Injuries in Assault Victims

TYPE	MECHANISM
Perioral or intraoral injuries, especially erythema/petechiae near junction of hard/soft palate	Hand restraint (voice muffling), forced penile-oral penetration
Neck bruises, "hickies"	Choke by hand or ligature, suction/bite
Oval or semicircular bruises to neck, chest, breasts, extremities	Bite
Impact bruises to face, body, especially lips and eyes; intra-abdominal hematomas or organ rupture	Penetrating blow with fist
Impact bruises to extensor surfaces of upper/lower arms, knuckles	Defense injuries (victim tries to protect head with arms)
Traumatic alopecia, subgaleal hematoma	Hair-pulling
Numerous small (2-3 cm) bruises on shoulders, arms, thighs, face	Hand restraint bruises or grab marks
Ligature marks to wrists/ankles	Restraint with rope or wire
Abrasions, friction injuries to bony prominences of back	Victim struggle while restrained in supine position on firm surface

adequate view of vulva, hymen, and vestibule. If hymen appears abnormal, examine in prone knee-chest position to confirm. In supine position, normal hymen can fold on itself, creating an artifactual abnormality of thickening or irregularity that unfolds on normalizes in prone position.

2. *Supine lithotomy position.* Used for larger prepubertal girls and all female adolescents. Feet placed in examination table stirrups, patient moves hips and buttocks to end of table and flexes knees outward to the side. Position provides adequate view of vulva, hymen, and vestibule.

3.   *Prone knee-chest position.* Used for prepubertal children and provides best view of perianal area (**Figure 7-1**). Child's shoulders, elbows, and forearms placed on table; lower back lordotic, extending hips upward; knees are placed about 18 inches apart. Important to confirm irregularities seen in supine position. With girls, position is helpful for confirming healed tears or clefts in hymen and possible to visualize vagina and cervix without inserting a speculum. With boys, penis and testicles are evaluated in supine position, but prone knee-chest position is helpful when looking for anorectal injury.

4.   *Supine knee-chest position.* Used for infants to examine anus. Lateral position may also be used. Knees are drawn up onto chest for visualization of perianal strictures.

5.   *Lateral decubitus position.* Used for all age groups to examine anus. Knees are together and drawn up onto chest so anus can be seen; avoid distortion of tissue with minimal gluteal separation (**Figures 7-2** and **7-3**).

— Approach:

1.   Tell the child you will explain everything before it happens.

2.   Raise the head of the examination table so the child can see you and you can gauge the child's reaction and anxiety level.

3.   Allow the child to change into examination gown in private and keep all other areas of body draped.

4.   Let the child choose a support person to be present during examination.

5.   Touch the child's knee or arm with sample cotton-tipped applicator before obtaining vaginal or anal cultures.

6.   When examining girls, begin with labial separation (move labia majora laterally and inferiorly), then progress to labial traction (grasp labial majora close to posterior commissure and pull gently in anterior direction).

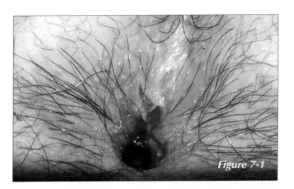

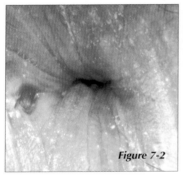
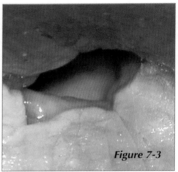

Figure 7-1. *Adolescent who denied anal penetration and denied any pain or bleeding in her anal area. In the prone knee-chest position, 2 tears are seen at 12 and 1 o'clock.*

Figure 7-2. *14-year-old girl with a history of anal penetration occurring 3 days prior. Note tear at 9 o'clock. Patient is in left lateral decubitus position.*

Figure 7-3. *15-year-old adolescent boy with a long-term history of anal-penile penetration. Note laxity of anal opening and scar tissue at 9 o'clock. Patient is in the lateral decubitus position.*

7.   Have the child assume lateral or prone knee-chest position as needed.

8.   Avoid shop talk during the examination.

9.   Move quickly and gently.

10. When using any of the examination techniques, apply constant, even, gentle pressure with fingers and avoid groping movements.

11. After the examination, have the child sit up or change into clothing before giving the results.

12. Discuss examination findings and treatment plans with the child or adolescent first, then caregivers, support adults, or investigators.

DOCUMENTING INJURIES

— During the genital examination, follow protocols for forensic evidence collection when indicated and then document genital and anal findings and test for STDs when appropriate.

— Photograph genital injuries with 35-mm camera equipped with ring flash and zoom lens or photocolposcope.

1. The photocolposcope may enhance detection of injuries when examination is done within 48 hours of vaginal-penile penetration.

2. Photographic documentation of injuries greatly enhances presentation of evidence in legal settings.

— Most sexual trauma victims have no visible anogenital injury.

1. Presence and extent of injury depend on various factors.

2. Acute injuries resolve completely within 1 to 5 days, though it depends on depth and location of injury.

3. An increased likelihood of visible injury exists if there is vaginal bleeding and if the examination is done within 72 hours of the assault (Adams et al, 1994).

— Injuries may be acute or healed.

1. Injuries from acute vaginal-penile penetration include lacerations (**Figures 7-4** and **7-5**), edema, and submucosal hemorrhages.

2. Most injuries occur in the posterior vestibule or posterior rim of hymen between 3 and 9 o'clock.

3. More severe injuries may extend to the perineum, lateral vestibule, and intravaginal area.

4. Genital trauma may be found even when a victim is asymptomatic.

5. Penetrating anal injuries also resolve rapidly and completely.

6. Acute anal findings include lacerations, hematomas, edema, and sphincter spasms.

7. Some anal or genital injuries take weeks to heal.

— Nonacute or healed injuries associated with vaginal penetration bear no legal significance in an adolescent with numerous sexual partners unless the victim has injuries caused by anal-penile penetration but no prior consensual contact of that nature.

1. Specifically ask whether anal-penile penetration occurred; many adolescents are reluctant to disclose this information unless asked directly.

2. Healed injuries include complete clefts of hymen (**Figures 7-6** and **7-7**) and scarring of the posterior vestibule or anus (**Figures 7-8** and **7-9**).

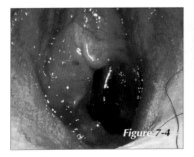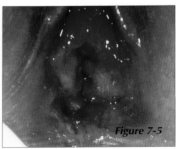

Figure 7-4. Hematoma. 15-year-old victim of vaginal-penile penetration 36 hours previously.

Figure 7-5. 5-year-old female victim of vaginal-penile penetration occurring 36 hours earlier. Complete hymenal tear at 6 o'clock, and posterior vestibule tear with bruising.

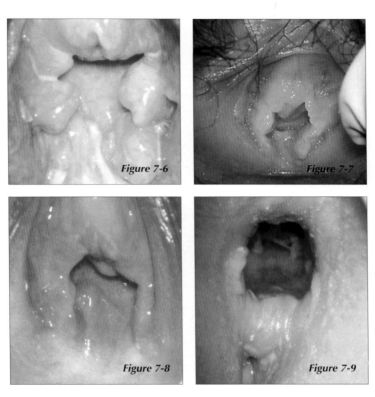

Figure 7-6. *Adolescent girl with several hymenal clefts, resulting in isolated "clumps" of hymen (caruncles). There is no visible hymenal tissue from 4 to 8 o'clock. History of long-term sexual activity with several individuals.*

Figure 7-7. *Healed tear, or cleft, from 5 to 7 o'clock.*

Figure 7-8. *Posterior vestibule scar and large area from 4 to 8 o'clock of no visible hymenal tissue.*

Figure 7-9. *13-year-old female victim of repeated anal-penile penetration by 2 individuals over a period of 3 to 4 years. Extensive perianal scarring and immediate anal sphincter dilatation is noted (patient is in the prone knee-chest position). The absence of stool in the anal vault and the presence of other traumatic findings supports trauma as the cause of this dilatation. The child also reported some difficulty with fecal incontinence over the past year.*

DIAGNOSTIC TESTING
STDs

— Child victims of pornography or prostitution should be comprehensively tested for STDs.

— Children and adolescents infected with STDs may or may not have symptoms.

1. Prepubertal girls with vaginal gonorrhea tend to be symptomatic (Siegel et al, 1995).

2. Adolescents with vaginal gonorrhea or chlamydia are less likely to have symptoms.

3. Herpes simplex virus (HSV) type 1 or 2 may occur on genitals or perianal tissues (**Figures 7-10** and **7-11**). Culture ulcerative or vesicular lesions for herpes. Definitive diagnosis is essential to appropriate long-term management and treatment.

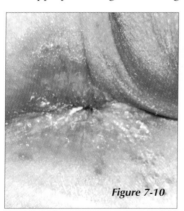
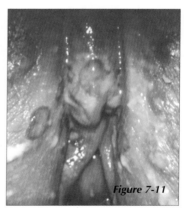

Figure 7-10. Herpes simplex virus (HSV) type 2 lesions with secondary Group A beta hemolytic streptococcus infection (note crusted leading edge, lower half of image) in a prepubertal girl with no history of sexual contact. She also had vaginal gonorrhea and chlamydia infections.

Figure 7-11. HSV type 1 in a 10-year-old girl who initially denied sexual contact. She later admitted to oral (perpetrator)-genital (victim) contact by a relative.

— The AAP (1991) recommends serum rapid plasma reagin (RPR) test; wet mount for *Trichomonas vaginalis*; throat, rectal, and genital cultures for *Neisseria gonorrhoeae*; and rectal and genital cultures for *Chlamydia trachomatis*.

— A positive test for STD is legally relevant only when a child or adolescent has had no sexual contact outside of the abuse.

— A sexually assaulted adolescent who has several sexual partners is at significant risk for STD and should be tested with the most sensitive detection techniques available.

— Centers for Disease Control and Prevention (CDC) (2002b) recommends nucleic acid amplification tests (NAATs), such as polymerase chain reaction (PCR) and ligase chain reaction tests for sexually active adults to detect *N gonorrhoeae* and *C trachomatis*.

— Examiners can submit a urine sample rather than a vaginal sample from adolescents who refuse examinations.

— Other diagnostic techniques for STDs include *Trichomonas* culture using InPouch TV, NAATs for HSV, and serological glycoprotein G–based assays for HSV-1 and HSV-2 (CDC, 2002a).

— Sexually active victims, victims of high-risk assault (multiple or unknown assailants), and victims who engage in other risky health behaviors should be tested for human immunodeficiency virus (HIV); hepatitis A (HAV), B (HBV), and C (HCV); and syphilis.

1. Acute disease can be diagnosed with serological confirmation of serum immunoglobulin M (IgM) antibody to HAV, IgM antibody to HBV core antigen, antibody to HCV, or HCV RNA (CDC, 2002a).

2. Positive RPR or Venereal Disease Reference Laboratory followed by positive treponemal-specific test (such as fluorescent treponemal antibody absorbed or *Treponema pallidum* particle agglutination) can confirm diagnosis of syphilis.

3. Some laboratories screen for syphilis with treponemal-specific enzyme-linked immunosorbent assay test; patients with positive

results are then tested with RPR to confirm active, untreated disease.

4. For HIV, begin with highly sensitive enzyme immunoassay, then confirm positive screens with Western blot or immunofluorescence assay for HIV antibodies. HIV antibody is detected in about 95% of patients within 3 months of infection (CDC, 2002a).

5. Serological testing during the initial visit and again 6 weeks later is recommended for HIV, syphilis, HAV, HBV, and HCV; serology for HIV should be repeated 12 and 24 weeks after initial testing.

6. Bacterial vaginosis is not conclusive of sexual transmission and can be diagnosed by wet mount examination (clue cells and leukocytosis).

7. Human papillomavirus infection (**Figures 7-12** and **7-13**) is usually diagnosed clinically or by Pap smear; a biopsy is needed only when lesions are atypical or do not resolve with treatment.

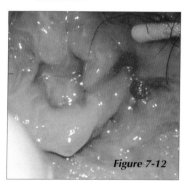 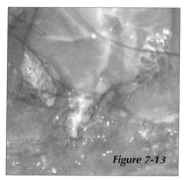

Figure 7-12. *Human papillomavirus (HPV) lesions (venereal warts) in an adolescent. Lesions at 3 o'clock were obscured by hymenal folds. Cotton-tipped applicator used to move hymenal flaps centrally in order to examine the vestibule for lesions.*

Figure 7-13. *HPV lesions in the posterior vestibule at 3, 6, and 9 o'clock.*

Pregnancy

— Do serum pregnancy testing before administering antimicrobial agents or pregnancy prophylaxis.

— Give emergency contraception only to nonpregnant girls.

— Because some evidence indicates oral contraceptives given during pregnancy may cause fetal abnormalities, consider this when prescribing estradiol and when counseling patients regarding its use.

Substance Abuse Screening/Testing/Monitoring

— Question all victims about drug and alcohol use.

— Test urine or serum for drugs only with patient's knowledge and consent or when mental status is compromised (Committee on Substance Abuse, 1998).

— Perform follow-up testing for monitoring purposes as part of treatment protocol.

Additional Laboratory Testing

— May reveal baseline liver function, thyroid status, bone growth, bone injury, and nutritional status.

DNA EVIDENCE PROCESSING AND ANALYSIS

— Processing usually requires weeks or months.

— Processing and analysis are expensive.

— Crime scene DNA profiles are examined with the intent to identify DNA from the victim or another person.

— Federal Bureau of Investigation can compare DNA profiles to those on file within the Combined DNA Index System (CODIS) database.

Methods of DNA Analysis

— *PCR of nuclear DNA*. Produces millions of copies of DNA so the archetype can be identified.

— *Restriction fragment length polymorphism*. Analysis of mitochondrial DNA; requires much larger sample.

— *PCR of mitochondrial DNA*. Used to identify samples not suitable for other 2 methods.

DNA Profiles Obtained

— *Inclusive.* Infers that an individual's DNA matches evidence from the crime scene. Reflects high likelihood that a person was present at a crime scene at some point in time.

— *Exclusive.* Suggests that the DNA profile generated from a crime scene does not match an individual.

— *Inconclusive.* Includes neither of other 2 possibilities.

COLLECTION AND STORAGE OF SPECIMENS

— Collect, transport, and preserve evidence in manner that resists contamination, intentional corruption, and degradation.

— Victims should not bathe, change clothes, douche, or wash hands.

— Authorities can examine and investigate a victim's space, but a trained sexual assault examiner must conduct physical examination of a victim's body.

— Conduct examinations as soon as possible to test for STDs and secure legitimate forensic evidence.

— Collection of DNA evidence usually requires a special kit.

— Contamination occurs as a result of handling without gloves, sneezing or coughing over specimen, exposure to heat and humidity, etc.

— Document the chain of custody to avoid corruption, loss, or theft.

TREATMENT

— Management of uncomplicated STDs is summarized in **Tables 7-10** and **7-11**.

FOLLOW-UP

— See **Table 7-12**.

— Make referrals as appropriate.

— Coordinate multidisciplinary long-term services for victims and supportive/nonabusive caregivers.

Table 7-10. Management of Uncomplicated Sexually Transmitted Diseases in Child* Victims of Sexual Abuse

Organism	Prophylactic Treatment	Treatment of Confirmed Disease
Gonorrhea	Cefixime 8 mg/kg (up to 400 mg) PO[†] x 1 or ceftriaxone 125 mg IM[†] x 1 PLUS treatment for chlamydia	Ceftriaxone 125 mg IM x 1
Chlamydia	Azithromycin 20 mg/kg (up to 1 g) PO x 1 or erythromycin 50 mg/kg/d x 10 days PLUS treatment for gonorrhea	Same as for prophylaxis
Hepatitis	Begin or complete hepatitis A and B immunization	None
Trichomonas, bacterial vaginitis	Consider: metronidazole 15 mg/d (TID[†]) x 7 days, or 40 mg/kg (up to 2 g) PO x 1	Same as for prophylaxis
Syphilis[‡]	Gonorrhea prophylaxis has efficacy against incubating syphilis	Benzathine penicillin G 50 000 U/kg IM x 1 up to 2.4 million U
Herpes simplex virus type 2	None	Acyclovir 80 mg/kg/d PO (TID-QID[†]) up to 1.0 g/d x 7-10 days
Human papillomavirus	None	Patient administered: podofilox 5% solution or gel or imiquimod 5% cream Clinician administered: podophyllin, trichloracetic acid, cryotherapy, or surgical excision
Human immuno-deficiency virus	No specific recommendations for children	Consult with infectious disease specialist

* *Preadolescent children weighing < 100 lbs.*
† *Abbreviations: PO=orally, IM=intramuscularly, TID=3 times daily, QID=4 times daily.*
‡ *Cerebrospinal fluid examination recommended prior to treating confirmed disease.*
Data from American Academy of Pediatrics, 2000.

Table 7-11. Management of Uncomplicated Sexually Transmitted Diseases in Adolescent* Victims of Sexual Abuse

Organism	Prophylactic Treatment	Treatment of Confirmed Disease
Gonorrhea	Cefixime 400 mg PO† x 1 or ceftriaxone 125 mg IM† x 1 PLUS treatment for chlamydia	Same as for prophylaxis
Chlamydia	Azithromycin 1 g PO x 1 PLUS treatment for gonorrhea	Azithromycin 1 g PO x 1 or doxycycline 200 mg/d (BID†) x 7 days
Hepatitis	Begin or complete hepatitis A and B immunization	None
Trichomonas, bacterial vaginosis	Metronidazole 2 g PO x 1	Metronidazole 2 g PO x 1 or 250 mg TID† x 7 days
Syphilis‡	Gonorrhea prophylaxis has efficacy against incubating syphilis	Benzathine penicillin G 2.4 million U IM x 1 or doxycycline 200 mg/d (BID) PO x 14 days
Herpes simplex virus type 2	None	Acyclovir 1000-1200 mg/d (3-5 x/d) PO x 7-10 d
Human papillomavirus	None	Patient administered: podofilox .5% solution or gel or imiquimod 5% cream Clinician administered: podophyllin, trichloracetic acid, cryotherapy, or surgical excision
Human immuno-deficiency virus	Consider if high-risk contact occurs: zidovudine 150 mg (BID) x 4 weeks	Consult with infectious disease specialist

* *Includes preadolescents weighing > 100 lbs.*
† *Abbreviations: PO=orally, IM=intramuscularly, BID=2 times daily, TID=3 times daily.*
‡ *Cerebrospinal examination is recommended for those with central nervous system symptoms.*
Data from American Academy of Pediatrics, 2000.

NORMAL ANATOMY

— Normal anatomic findings divide childhood into 3 phases:

1. *Infant or toddler*. Children between birth and 5 years of age; normally no endogenous estrogen effect in girls

2. *Juvenile or preadolescent*. Immature and prepubescent boys and girls (usually before menarche) aged 6 to 12 years

3. *Adolescent*. Boys and postpubertal, menstruating, and childbearing girls aged 13 to 18 years

— Important aspects include landmarks, gross vascularity, and neurological innervations.

Table 7-12. Follow-Up Considerations for Victims of Sexual Trauma

2 Weeks

— Healing of injuries

— Type 2 herpes simplex virus: 3-10 days' incubation

— Trichomoniasis, bacterial vaginosis, chlamydia, gonorrhea: 10-14 days' incubation (if no initial prophylaxis given)

— Pregnancy (if oral contraception is not provided at initial evaluation)

— Psychological support/reassurance

— Drug/alcohol monitoring/treatment (if coordinated with specialist)

2-3 Months

— HIV testing: repeat at 6 weeks, 3 months, 6 months, 1 year

— Syphilis and hepatitis: 6-8 weeks' incubation

— Human papillomavirus: 2-3 months' average incubation; up to 20 months' incubation in rare cases

— Psychological support

— Drug/alcohol monitoring (if coordinated with specialist)

Adapted from Kellogg & Sugarek, 1998.

— Changes in male and female children reflect hormonal alterations and physical growth (Berenson, 1998).

NORMAL GENITALIA

Boys

— Determine penile length, foreskin anatomy, urethral meatus location, scrotal anatomy (darkening and enlargement), presence and/or absence of testes, scrotal hair growth, presence and/or absence of scrotal or inguinal masses.

— Examine upper urinary components.

— Perform scrotal transillumination with a bright, cool light source to identify lack of testicular descent.

— Without circumcision, foreskin retraction occurs by the age of 5 years; careful examination may differentiate trauma from balanitis and phimosis.

— Male development approaching age 11 to 12 years:

1. First sign of pubertal onset is testicular growth and/or enlargement.

2. Pubic hair is visible.

3. Penile length, hair growth, testicular size increase throughout puberty and adolescence.

4. Race influences anatomy (Kadish et al, 1998).

— Injuries to male urethra caused by physical violence cause urethral rupture near the prostate gland.

1. Urine extravasates into perineum, shaft of penis swells, and perineum in front of anus and scrotal sac distends.

2. Swelling can ascend into abdominal wall.

— Scrotum, testes, and penis derive predominant nerve supply from lumbar nerves 10 and 11 and sacral nerves 2 through 4.

— Blood supply derives from internal and external pudendal arteries and veins, tributaries of the internal iliac artery and veins.

Girls

— Findings in neonatal girl in supine position with legs flexed:

1. Separation of labia reveals clitoris, vaginal introitus, hymen, and urethral meatus.

2. Follicles in fossa navicularis, periurethral bands, labial adhesions, vestibular erythema, fourchette avascularity, and urethral dilation are normal, nonabusive findings.

3. Consider imperforate hymen, foul vaginal discharge, retained foreign body before assuming sexual abuse (Botash & Jean-Louis, 2001).

— Hymenal findings (**Figures 7-14-a, b, c, d,** and **e**):

1. *Newborns.* Redundant, thick, and estrogenized because of in utero exposure to maternal hormones (Berenson et al, 1991).

2. *Prepubertal.* Annular, crescentic, thin, redundant, cuff-like, and unestrogenized hymen (Berenson et al, 1992).

3. *Pubertal.* Thick, elastic, estrogenized hymen from an endogenous source (Heger et al, 2002).

4. White discharge is common at all ages.

5. Imperforate, cribriform, septate, and microperforate hymen configurations reflect congenital abnormalities or other etiologies to be clinically excluded.

— Examination position of infants and neonates is similar, with the perivaginal skin in posterolateral fashion. Findings in infants will be different than neonates because they lack in utero exposure to maternal hormones.

— Findings in preadolescent patients, frog-leg or knee-chest position:

1. At puberty, breast development is followed by pubic hair growth.

2. Vaginal mucosa lacks estrogen and is thin and reddened with a watery, non–foul-smelling discharge.

3. Vagina is estrogen-stimulated, with elasticity and thickening.

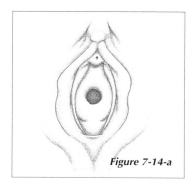

Figure 7-14-a

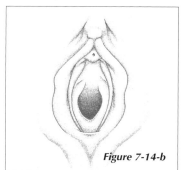

Figure 7-14-b

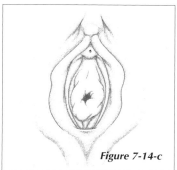

Figure 7-14-c

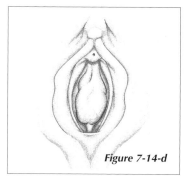

Figure 7-14-d

Figures 7-14-a, b, c, d, and **e.** Types of hymen include annular (a), crescentic (b), cuff-like (c), imperforate (d), and septate (e).

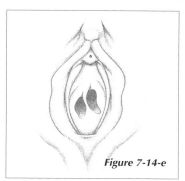

Figure 7-14-e

4. Leukorrhea (nonfoul watery discharge) is normal.

5. Blood, foul discharge, or odor requires further investigation.

6. Other cases:

    A. External vaginal soft-tissue masses in girls represent urethral prolapse with eversion (young African American girls in particular).

    B. Lichen sclerosis, a rare skin disorder that mimics abusive trauma, may manifest as ulcers, fissures, or hypertrophy of the perianal skin.

    C. Coincidental genital trauma is situational and found with consensual sex, with or without pregnancy, and in nonsexual physical assault (Jones et al, 2003).

— Female circumcision:

1. It is also called *female genital mutilation* (FGM) or *female genital cutting*.

2. It is a cross-cultural, cross-religious ritual that refers to removal of portions of the female external genitalia (American College of Obstetricians and Gynecologists, 1999; Aziz, 1980; *Female Genital Mutilation*, 1997; Toubia, 1994, 1995).

3. Girls may be circumcised as young as age 3 years.

4. **Figure 7-15** shows normal female genitalia; **Figures 7-16-a, b,** and **c** show various types of FGM procedures.

Differential Diagnosis of Genital Trauma

— Speculum examination with cervical visualization is not appropriate for prepubertal children unless done under anesthesia, though it may be appropriate in adolescents.

— To successfully diagnose certain childhood conditions, consider using imaging technologies.

— For chronic injuries that prompt emergency clinical questions, use interventional radiology.

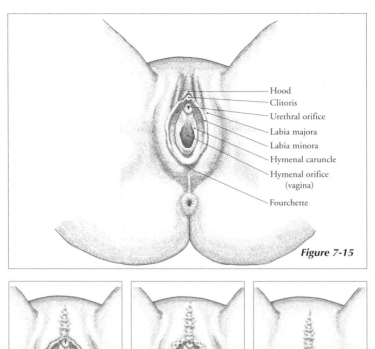

Hood
Clitoris
Urethral orifice
Labia majora
Labia minora
Hymenal caruncle
Hymenal orifice
(vagina)
Fourchette

Figure 7-15

Figure 7-16-a

Figure 7-16-b

Figure 7-16-c

Figure 7-15. Normal female genitalia.

Figures 7-16-a, b, and *c.* Type I (a), type II (b), and type III (c) procedures of female circumcision.

— Laparoscopy is liberally applied to address pain syndromes and intra-abdominal injury.

— Vaginal bleeding (Emans, 1998):

1. Prepubertal girl: trauma, vulvovaginitis, endocrine abnormalities, dermatoses, condyloma accuminata, foreign body, urethral prolapse, blood dyscrasia, hemangioma, tumor

2. Adolescent girl: anovulatory uterine bleeding, pregnancy-related complications, infection, blood dyscrasias, endocrine disorders, vaginal abnormalities (carcinoma, laceration), cervical problems, uterine problems, ovarian problems (cyst, tumor), endometriosis, trauma, foreign body, systemic diseases, medications

DETERMINING AGE IN CHILD PORNOGRAPHY

— Child pornography, also often referred to as child sexual abuse images, is the depiction of a crime scene. When determining the likely ages of children victimized in this manner, the key points of analysis include:

1. An objective analysis of what is shown in the image, avoiding speculation as to how the image might have been altered to appear that way.

2. The corresponding file name, which often accurately reflects the image content.

3. Whether the image is consistent with a child younger than the legal age guidelines cited in a state or federal statute (eg, younger than 12 years or younger than 18 years).

4. The degree of sexual abuse is depicted in the image (eg, digital molestation of 1 child by another versus sadistic sexual abuse).

Musculoskeletal Development

— Order radiographic studies to determine bone age. Use accepted standards that measure maturation of the carpal bones in the hands.

— Head height and total height ratio comparisons compare crown-to-chin height with total height (crown to sole of foot). Typical results:

1. *Toddlers*. Ratio of 1:5.

2. *School-aged children (aged 5 to 7 years)*. Ratio of 1:6.

3. *Young persons (aged 15 years)*. Approximate ratio of 1:6.5.

4. *Adults*. Ratio of 1:7.5 or 1:8.

— Use adjunct analysis with caution in pornographic images because images may have become distorted with use of programs that allow morphological changes. A computer-based image does not always provide an examiner with opportunity to fully assess a child's height because the body may not be fully exposed.

— Other considerations: actual muscular development (muscular development of pectoralis muscles as androgens and estrogens become more available with maturation); pubertal growth spurt in boys; body habitus changes in boys (eg, shoulders broadening); hormonal influences that affect the pubertal process and physical manifestations.

Dental Maturation

— When mandibular maturation begins, children begin to shed their teeth.

— Central incisors of the mandible are usually lost at age 6 to 7 years, maxillary front teeth at age 7 to 8 years.

— New eruption of permanent teeth usually occurs almost immediately after deciduous shedding.

— If a child has missing canines and larger, secondary central incisors are present, the examiner can reasonably conclude the child is 9 to 11 years of age.

— Malnutrition is associated with advanced tooth shedding, but there should be more evidence of malnutrition than just dental findings.

ASSESSMENT OF A CHILD'S ETHNICITY

— The most reliable ancestry assignment is made with the adult skull, with the 3 most discernible skull differences found in those of Asian, African, and European descent.

— When a cadaver is discovered, determination of ancestry is important to facilitate identification of the body.

— Forensic anthropologists establish ancestry either by osteological discernable differences or osteometry.

1. *Anthroposcopy*. Entails the use of visually discernible differences noted in the skull's shape and the orientation of facial features.

2. *Osteometry*. Uses metric measurements to compare a known victim to standard measurements within a culture.

— Visual review of the living human face requires far less knowledge than that of forensic pathology and anthropology.

1. Racial differences are often more than just skin pigmentation. The shape of the eyes, the appearance of the hair, and often the nasal form qualities assist an examiner when establishing ancestry.

2. Examiners acknowledge that few pure ethnic groups exist. Interracial/interethnic mixing over generations makes the establishment of ancestry based solely on visual facial features not completely accurate. See also Chapter 9, Investigating Child Pornography.

Assessing Toddler Pornography

— Child pornography collections show victims as young as infants, toddlers, or preschool-aged children (younger than 60 months).

— Medical examiners can assess a child's gross motor skills to help identify the child's developmental level (see also Chapter 9, Investigating Child Pornography).

1. Toddlers who walk with their hands above their head (referred to as high-guard gait) or at shoulder level (mid-guard gait) are just beginning to walk independently.

2. A high-guard and mid-guard hand stance is usually associated with a wide-based foot placement with each step, attesting to the child's lack of integration of motor skills.

3. When this pattern is seen, the child is aged 13 to 15 months.

4.   Developing the normal, reciprocating swing of the arms is affected by prematurity, motor strength, cognition, and general neurological tone (Bly, 1994).

5.   Toddlers tend to develop the skill of walking backward while pulling an object between ages 12.5 and 20 months. The skill is comparable to facing forward and using one hand to pull an object behind the body, which develops at about 15 months and is mastered by 18 months.

6.   The average age of a child who can carry a large object while walking is 17 to 18.5 months.

7.   Children can squat while playing normally at about age 20 to 21 months.

SEXUAL MATURATION

— Often child pornography depicts youths with various degrees of sexual maturation but who do not appear to be completely sexually mature. The transition through puberty usually entails 4 to 6 years of physical development.

— Sexual maturation assessments should be stated as sexual maturation ratings and follow the accepted designations of B (breast development), PH (pubic hair distribution), and G (gonad development). Because visual depictions are being evaluated, practical assessments only include breast and pubic hair determinations.

— Additional physical aspects of adolescent development include axillary hair, acne, muscle development, general habitus with shoulder, waist, and hip appearances, and the presence of facial and perianal hair.

— References regarding the age norms for sexual maturation ratings for youths in the United States based upon racial groups (blacks, whites, and Hispanics) can be found via the Third National Health and Nutrition Examination Survey (NHANES III) and Pediatric Research in Office Settings (PROS).

1. On average, full sexual maturation based on breast and pubic hair growth for girls is approximately achieved by the ages of 14 years (black), 15 years (white), and 16 years (Mexican American).

2. Boys of all 3 races average physical sexual maturation between the ages of 15 and 16 years, with the majority reaching this milestone before the age of 16 years.

— It is imperative to avoid the use of the Tanner stage designations when discussing child pornography because of an opinion stated by Drs Arlan Rosenbloom and James Tanner that the original stages should not be cited for this purpose (1998).

INJURIES SPECIFIC TO THE SEXUAL EXPLOITATION OF CHILDREN

DIAGNOSING RAPE

— In infants, rape is diagnosed for any established contact for sexual stimulation (Resnick et al, 2000).

— Rape diagnoses become more difficult to ascertain as children grow older.

DIAGNOSING PHYSICAL INJURIES

— Genital injury related to the sexual exploitation of children may not always produce visible physical evidence. It may not be apparent during examination of child's genitals if the assault occurred more than 72 hours before the examination.

— Injury occurs less often in chronic cases (American Academy of Pediatrics, Committee on Child Abuse and Neglect, 1991).

— There are many variables related to the degree of injury to the victim.

1. Certain perpetrator characteristics are related to degree of injury, such as age, motive for injury, and relationship of the offender to the child.

2. Family members tend to inflict less injury and use more intimidation.

3. Unknown assailants tend to ensure a greater chance of injury and are more likely to use threats of injury or death.

— Forced penetration is often evidenced by tears in and around the vagina or anus.

1. Tears can occur secondary to hematoma-induced expansion.

2. Healed lacerations or tears in introitus may manifest with hymenal changes, which are chronicled by diameters and locations of disruptions or ridges (McCann et al, 1992).

3. Erythema is an often-transient and obscure finding. Sexual assault experts are attuned to recognize abrasions and redness.

4. Fistula formation usually occurs after healing and may reflect chronic assault. This requires a fluent knowledge of normal age-specific anatomy (Adams et al, 1992).

— Sexual maturity of children is reflected in many body sites.

1. Precocious puberty may result in changes of voice, hair, skin texture, and breasts plus other subtle changes.

2. Putting genital findings in context emphasizes the need for well-trained and experienced sexual assault assessment team to adequately gauge the extent and impact of genital injury.

— Injuries are generally classified as *visible* or *physical* (Elam & Ray, 1986) and *invisible* or *inoculation* (eg, viral inoculation such as herpes simplex or human papillomavirus).

1. Determining whether an injury is invisible or inoculated requires serial visits, examinations, and laboratory testing at the time of injury (Slaughter et al, 1997).

2. Forecasting the victim's subsequent reproductive future is futile because of possible inoculation injuries.

3. Physical and laboratory evaluation of an alleged perpetrator is an inadequate predictor of inoculation injuries in victim (Muram, 1989).

— When reevaluating a child during a follow-up examination, first review all laboratory results from the initial postassault examination, including written medical and forensic evidence.

— Next, complete physical examination, beginning with a whole-body examination and followed by a genital examination.

Management

Acute Visible Injuries

— Visible injuries, such as lacerations or tears, may require suture repair.

— If hemorrhage is controllable, apply ice and pressure (Sachs & Chu, 2002).

— Vagina may have first-, second-, third-, or fourth-degree lacerations ranging from simple epithelial disruption of the vagina or perineum to the complete division of rectal sphincter and rectal mucosal tear.

— Estrogen mediated distensibility of the vagina influences the degree of laceration and bleeding.

— Manage first- or second-degree injuries conservatively; third- and fourth-degree injuries require suture repair to align the structures in an anatomically correct fashion and secure function (Berenson et al, 2000).

— Hematomas may manifest with expansion that necessitates incision and drainage.

1. Take care not to compromise the underlying visceral blood supply to the uterus, bladder, or bowel.

2. Use general anesthetic to ensure patient compliance without compromising the appropriate resistance.

3. Deep-vessel injury may necessitate exploration of the abdominal cavity to expunge adjacent visceral injury (Adams, 1996).

— Genital injuries to boys that require significant suturing should be handled by general surgeon or urologist. Intervention may entail exploration, cauterization, packing for tamponade, suturing, or drainage (active and passive).

ACUTE INTERNAL INJURIES
To Reproductive Organs
— Degree of injury to internal reproductive organs is contingent on extent of abdominal trauma.

1. A great deal of force must be transmitted to cause internal pelvic injury.

2. The abdominal wall absorbs much energy and is usually bruised or lacerated.

3. Internal injury can occur as a result of severe physical trauma or an indolent inoculation insult.

4. Some STDs infect only the cervix, but unabated, these diseases can attack the fallopian tubes. The offending organism ascends from the vagina, through the cervix, out of the tubes, and into the peritoneal cavity. This syndrome, called pelvic inflammatory disease (PID), can manifest with the involvement of the pelvic peritoneum by inflammation and pus, adhesions, and tubal obstruction if left untreated. Subsequent pregnancies may put patients at risk for ectopic implantation.

— Laboratory tests with serial complete blood counts, urinalysis, cervical cultures, and imaging by ultrasound and/or computed tomography (CT) scan provide objective signs of progress or lack thereof.

— Laparoscopy and laparotomy are also possible treatment options for resistant cases of PID.

1. Laparoscopy allows serial bacterial dilution with simple saline or lactated Ringer's solution, thereby decreasing the infectious load, augmenting the antibiotic effect, and shortening the recovery period.

2. Hysterectomy with the removal of the fallopian tubes and ovaries is an option for the worst-case scenarios.

To Bony Pelvis
— The bony pelvis, or the fracture of the bony perimeter, is another internal injury that may occur when a victim is struck by a vehicle,

thrown from a moving vehicle or a building, or struck with a blunt object as might be seen in a case associated with sexual exploitation through prostitution.

— Definitive diagnosis may require a radiograph or CT scan, though magnetic resonance imaging offers the most reliable visualization.

— Immobilization is a rare treatment option, since venous thrombosis is a major potential complication.

— Orthopedic consultation is recommended.

— Soft-tissue injury and damage is expected in these cases; therefore, serial general surgical evaluations are required.

PSYCHIATRIC EMERGENCIES

— Actively suicidal or psychotic patients need hospitalization, observation, and an evaluation for medication.

— These patients may be managed by a psychiatric consultant.

— Screen for substance abuse in all suicidal, homicidal, and psychotic patients.

SADISTIC ABUSE OF INFANTS/TODDLERS

— This degree of abuse has significant effects because penile-vaginal penetration at this age is extremely painful and results in direct tissue trauma.

— Anal penetration can harm the child physically and psychologically, depending on the size of the penetrating object.

— Infants who have been penetrated may be preverbal, but pain management studies reveal that infants perceive pain as acutely as adults, meaning that blood pressure, heart rate, diaphoresis, and distress all increase.

— Sexual and physical abuse of young children influences developing brain neuroarchitecture, causing cellular and structural changes in the limbic system, with lifelong impact (eg, posttraumatic stress disorder) (Teicher et al, 2002, 2003).

FORENSIC EVIDENCE COLLECTION

— Recovery of forensic evidence among postpubertal patients is higher than in prepubertal children due to physiologic differences and the fact that more adolescents may seek treatment within a time frame conducive to evidence collection.

— Children's clothing is much more productive of forensic evidence as compared to their skin.

— Foreign material, head hair combings/pluckings, clothing, and debris should be collected first.

1. Debris or foreign bodies found in the mouth, vagina, or rectum are submitted as evidence.

2. Pubic hair combings/pluckings and swabs from the mouth, vagina, or rectum are submitted for analysis.

3. Patient saliva and blood samples are also required to establish the patient's blood type and whether blood group antigens were secreted into bodily fluids.

— Evidence collection follows protocols established by state or regional crime laboratories; maintain chain of custody for collected material (see also Chapters 11, Investigating Cyber-Enticement, 12, Legal Issues Specific to Pornography Cases, and 13, Legal Considerations in Prostitution Cases).

SEX OFFENDER ASSESSMENTS

— Assessments have gained new importance in the prosecution and treatment of male offenders.

— Consequences are always serious, especially given the frequency with which sex offender assessment results are introduced during the sentencing phase of judicial hearings.

— Most professionals who conduct such assessments appear to do so thoughtfully and ethically after taking part in the substantial training needed to work with this select clinical population.

STANDARDS AND GUIDELINES

— Standards of the Association for the Treatment of Sexual Abusers (ATSA) are considered the best standards for psychosexual evaluations.

— Sex offender assessments should include information in distinct areas of behavior and functioning (**Table 7-13**).

— Sources for assessment information include client interviews, self-report measures or psychometric tests, interviews with collateral informants, psychophysiological testing, and review of official documents.

MEASURES USED

— Physiological measure of sexual arousal and interest: penile plethysmography (**Figure 7-17**).

1. It is adapted from volumetric plethysmograph that uses a strain gauge.

2. It is used by 25% to 34% of adult community and residential treatment programs (McGrath et al, 2003).

3. It is the single best predictor of recidivism risk in child molesters (Hanson & Bussiere, 1998).

4. Principal ethical concerns stem from previously common use of nude stimuli, inappropriate application of plethysmography to certain populations, and inappropriate interpretations of data.

— Measurement of dissimulation:

1. *Current viewing time (VT).* Developed to avoid specific concerns with plague ple-

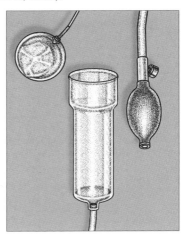

Figure 7-17. *Volumetric plethysmograph.*

thysmography testing. Based on length of time subjects view slides of models who differ in age and gender (Abel et al, 1998).

Table 7-13. Information to Be Obtained in All Psychosexual Evaluations

— Availability of appropriate community supports

— Access to potential victims

— Criminal and other antisocial behavior and values

— Developmental history and family background

— Deviant sexual interests and arousal

— Education and employment histories

— History of aggression or violence

— History of sexually abusive behavior, including details about victims, tactics used in the commission of the offense, and the circumstances in which the sexual abuse occurred

— Insight into offense precursors and risk

— Level of cognitive functioning and other responsivity factors

— Level of self-disclosure and accountability

— Medical and mental health history

— Official and unreported history of sexual and nonsexual crimes

— Peer and romantic relationship history

— Relevant personality traits such as, but not limited to suspiciousness, hostility, risk-taking, impulsivity, and psychopathy

— Sexual history, including sexual fantasies, urges, and behavior, early sexual experiences; number and duration of sexual relationships; gender identity and sexual orientation; masturbation and intercourse frequency; sexual functioning; and unusual sexual interests or behavior that are not sexually deviant or illegal, such as cross-gender dressing

— Substance use

— Use of sexually arousing materials (eg, magazines, computer pornography, books, videos, Internet sites, telephone sex services)

Reprinted with permission from section D.19 from the Association for the Treatment of Sexual Abusers, 2005.

Highly standardized; includes only nonnude stimuli. Principal ethical concerns stem from misinterpretation of VT results and use of measure with subjects from understudied populations.

2. *Polygraphy*. Ethical issues generated sufficient interest so that specific recommendations for its use with sex offenders were developed (Wilcox, 2000; ATSA, 2001). Concerns based on limited theory upon which polygraph testing is based, difficulty in testing validity of polygraph due to inherent difficulty ascertaining actual truth regarding any given question, and application of polygraph to situations where there is limited evidence of validity.

— Measurement of psychopathy: The Hare Psychopathy Checklist.

1. It is more discriminating conceptually and methodologically, with greater predictive validity.

2. Psychopathy is defined as personality disorder and describes individuals who are callous, lack empathy, and engage in destructive behaviors with no apparent concern for the rights of others.

3. Ethical issues concern appropriate training of examiners and application of personality diagnoses to minors.

— Conditions contributing to the likelihood of misinterpretation:

1. Assessments conducted before findings of guilt

2. Evaluations performed in the absence of guilty pleas

3. Assessments conducted with vulnerable subjects (minors and mentally retarded/developmentally delayed clients)

— Why conduct testing:

1. Pragmatic reasons; the cost of examination is covered by judicial system if client agrees to participate before adjudication.

2. Defense lawyer may want to have a more complete picture of client.

3. The results can be used in defense or prosecution.

REFERENCES

Abel GG, Huffman J, Warberg B, Holland CL. Visual reaction time and plethysmography as measures of sexual interest in child molesters. *Sex Abuse.* 1998;10:81-96.

Adams JA. Evolution of a classification scale: medical evaluation of suspected child sexual abuse. *Child Maltreat.* 2001;6:31-36.

Adams JA. Medical evaluation of suspected child sexual abuse. In: Pokorny SF, ed. *Pediatric and Adolescent Gynecology.* New York, NY: Chapman & Hall; 1996:1-14.

Adams JA, Harper K, Knudson S. A proposed system for the classification of anogenital findings in children with suspected sexual abuse. *Adolesc Pediatr Gynecol.* 1992;5:73-75.

Adams JA, Harper K, Knudson S, Revilla J. Examination findings in legally confirmed child sexual abuse: it's normal to be normal. *Pediatrics.* 1994;94(3):310-317.

American Academy of Pediatrics. *2000 Red Book: Report of the Committee on Infectious Diseases.* 25th ed. Elk Grove Village, Ill: American Academy of Pediatrics; 2000.

American Academy of Pediatrics Committee on Child Abuse and Neglect. Guidelines for the evaluation of sexual abuse of children. *Pediatrics.* 1991;87:254-260.

American Academy of Pediatrics Committee on Child Abuse and Neglect. Guidelines for the evaluation of sexual abuse of children. *Pediatrics.* 1999;103(1):186-191.

American Academy of Pediatrics, C. Henry Kempe National Center on Child Abuse and Neglect. *The Visual Diagnosis of Child Physical Abuse.* Elk Grove Village, Ill: American Academy of Pediatrics; 1994.

American College of Obstetricians and Gynecologists (ACOG). *Female Circumcision/Female Genital Mutilation: Clinical Management of Circumcised Women* [slide-lecture kit]. Washington, DC: ACOG; 1999.

Association for the Treatment of Sexual Abusers (ATSA). *Practice Standards and Guidelines for Members of the Association for the Treatment of Sexual Abusers*. Portland, Ore: ATSA; 2001:8.

Association for the Treatment of Sexual Abusers (ATSA). *Practice Standards and Guidelines for Members of the Association for the Treatment of Sexual Abusers*. Portland, Ore: ATSA; 2005:13-14.

Aziz FA. Gynecologic and obstetric complications of female circumcision. *Int J Gynaecol Obstet*. 1980;17:560-563.

Berenson AB, Chacko MR, Wiemann CM, Mishaw CO, Friedrich WN, Grady JJ. A case control study of anatomic changes resulting from sexual abuse. *Am J Obstet Gynecol*. 2000;182:820-831.

Berenson AB, Heger AH, Andrews S. Appearance of the hymen in newborns. *Pediatrics*. 1991;87:458-465.

Berenson AB, Heger AH, Hayes JM, Bailey RK, Emans SJ. Appearance of the hymen in prepubertal girls. *Pediatrics*. 1992;89:387-394.

Berenson AB. Normal anogenital anatomy. *Child Abuse Negl*. 1998; 22:589-596.

Bly L. *Motor Skills Acquisition in the First Year: An Illustrated Guide to Normal Development*. San Antonio, Tex: The Psychological Corporation; 1994.

Botash AS, Jean-Louis F. Imperforate hymen: congenital or acquired from sexual abuse? *Pediatrics*. 2001;109:e53.

CeASAR: The Center for Adolescent Substance Abuse Research. The CRAFFT questions. Available at: http://www.slp3d2.com/rwj_1027/webcast/docs/screentest.html. Accessed July 29, 2003.

Centers for Disease Control and Prevention. Screening tests to detect *Chlamydia trachomatis* and *Neisseria gonorrhoeae* infections. *MMWR Recomm Rep*. 2002a;51:1-38.

Centers for Disease Control and Prevention. Sexually transmitted diseases treatment guidelines. *MMWR Recomm Rep*. 2002b;51(No. RR-6):1-80.

Committee on Substance Abuse, American Academy of Pediatrics. Tobacco, alcohol, and other drugs: the role of the pediatrician in prevention and management of substance abuse. *Pediatrics.* 1998; 101(1):125-128.

Elam AL, Ray VG. Sexually related trauma: a review. *Ann Emerg Med.* 1986;15:576-584.

Emans SJ. Vulvovaginal problems in the prepubertal child. In: Emans SJ, Laufer MR, Goldstein DP, eds. *Pediatric and Adolescent Gynecology.* 4th ed. Philadelphia, Pa: Lippencott-Raven; 1998:75-107.

Female Genital Mutilation: A Joint WHO/UNICEF/UNFPA Statement. Geneva, Switzerland: World Health Organization; 1997.

Fishman M, Bruner A, Adger H. Substance abuse among children and adolescents. *Pediatr Rev.* 1997;18:394-403.

Hanson RK, Bussier MT. Predicting relapse: a meta-analysis of sexual offender recidivism studies. *J Consult Clin.* 1998;66:348-362.

Heger A, Emans SJ, eds. *Evaluation of the Sexually Abused Child: A Medical Textbook and Photographic Atlas.* New York, NY: Oxford University Press; 1992.

Heger AH, Ticson L, Guerra L, et al. Appearance of the genitalia in girls selected for nonabuse: review of hymenal morphology and nonspecific findings. *J Pediatr Adolesc Gynecol.* 2002;15:27-35.

Jones JS, Rossman L, Hartmann M, Alexander CC. Anogenital injuries in adolescents after consensual sexual intercourse. *Acad Emerg Med.* 2003;10:1378-1383.

Kadish HA, Schunk JE, Britton H. Pediatric male rectal and genital trauma: accidental and nonaccidental injuries. *Pediatr Emerg Care.* 1998;14:95-98.

Kellogg ND, Sugarek NJ. Sexual trauma. *Atlas of Office Procedures.* 1998;1:181-197.

Lenahan LC, Ernst A, Johnson B. Colposcopy in evaluation of the adult sexual assault victim. *Am J Emerg Med.* 1998;16:183-184.

McCann J, Voris J, Simon M. Genital injuries resulting from sexual abuse: a longitudinal study. *Pediatrics*. 1992;89:307-317.

McGrath RJ, Cumming GF, Burchard BL. *Current Practices and Trends in Sexual Abuser Management: the Safer Society 2002 Nationwide Survey*. Brandon, Vt: The Safer Society Foundation; 2003.

Muram D. Child sexual abuse: relationship between sexual acts and genital findings. *Child Abuse Negl*. 1989;13:211-216.

Neinstein LS, Ratner Kaufman F. Normal physical growth and development. In: Neinstein LS, ed. *Adolescent Health Care: A Practical Guide*. 4th ed. Philadelphia, Pa: Lippincott Williams & Wilkins; 2002:50-55.

Patel M, Minshall L. Management of sexual assault.*merg Med Clin North Am*. 2001;19:817-831.

Resnick H, Acierno R, Holmes M, Dammeyer M, Kilpatrick D. Emergency evaluation and intervention with female victims of rape and other violence. *J Clin Psychol*. 2000;56:1317-1333.

Rosenbloom AL, Tanner JM. Misuse of Tanner puberty stages to estimate chronologic age. *Pediatrics*. 1998;102:1494.

Sachs CJ, Chu LD. Predictors of genitorectal injury in female victims of suspected sexual assault. *Acad Emerg Med*. 2002;9:146-151.

Schwartz B, Alderman EM. Substances of abuse. *Pediatr Rev*. 1997; 18:204-215.

Siegel RM, Schubert CJ, Myers PA, Shapiro RA. The prevalence of sexually transmitted diseases in children and adolescents evaluated for sexual abuse in Cincinnati: rationale for limited STD testing on prepubertal girls. *Pediatrics*. 1995;96(6):1090-1094.

Slaughter L, Brown CR, Crowley S, Peck R. Patterns of genital injury in female sexual assault victims. *Am J Obstet Gynecol*. 1997;176:609-616.

Teicher MH, Andersen SI, Polcari A, Anderson CM, Navalta CP: Developmental neurobiology of childhood stress and trauma. *Psychiatr Clin North Am*. 2002;25(2):397-426.

Teicher MH, Andersen SL, Polcari A, Anderson CM, Navalta CP, Kim DM. The neurobiological consequences of early stress and childhood maltreatment. *Neurosci Biobehav Rev.* 2003;27(1-2):33-44.

Toubia N. Female circumcision as a public health issue. *N Engl J Med.* 1994;331:712-716.

Toubia N. *Female Genital Mutilation: A Call for Global Action.* New York, NY: RAINBO; 1995.

Unger JB, Simon TR, Newman TL, Montgomery SB, Kipke MD, Albornoz M. Early adolescent street youth: an overlooked population with unique problems and service needs. *J Early Adolesc.* 1998; 18(4):325-349.

Wilcox DT. Application of the clinical polygraph examination to the assessment, treatment, and monitoring of sex offenders. *Sex Aggress.* 2000;5:134-152, 138.

Chapter

PRINCIPLES OF INVESTIGATION

Det Sgt Joseph S. Bova Conti, BA
Michelle K. Collins, MA
Katherine A. Free, MA
Col Thomas P. O'Connor, BA, MA
Raymond C. Smith
Govind Prasad Thapa, MA, BL, MPA, PhD

— The investigation of child sexual exploitation (CSE) requires knowledge, skills, sensitivity, and a particular aptitude.

— Male and female investigators require special training to meet the needs of victims with professionalism and competence.

— The collection of facts and evidence is essential to all investigations, but special attention must be paid to:

1. Collecting preliminary information and data about the case to determine which way an investigation should proceed.

2. Showing considerable sensitivity to the victim's psychosocial status.

— The process begins as soon as a case is reported or, as in many trafficking cases when no one reports the case, when a victim is rescued or released.

PRELIMINARY INVESTIGATION BY FIRST RESPONDERS

— First responders are usually uniformed officers. They are responsible for evaluating the situation and taking the first investigative steps.

— Begin with and base the investigation on a well-documented account of all observations, actions, parties present, and evidence relevant to the scene.

1. Compile facts and ideas to determine whether a crime was committed and, if possible, who is responsible.

2. Make the critical link between mere suspicion and formal accusation.

— Factors in the preliminary investigative process:

1. Upon arriving at the scene, start recording observations.

    A. Include visual observations and details about what is being said.

    B. Note anything relevant that is said spontaneously.

2. Immediately determine whether the victim needs medical assistance and initiate needed procedures to provide care (see Chapter 7, Medical Issues).

3. Identify and interview all witnesses. Note the involvement of each in the incident.

4. Establish a timeline detailing who, what, where, when, how, and why. This document becomes the worksheet for the investigation.

5. Find and appropriately seize physical evidence.

    A. If necessary, obtain the suspect's consent before searching for evidence.

    B. Recognize potential evidence and take the steps needed to preserve it.

    C. Remember the complexities of electronic imaging and associated technical equipment.

    D. Remember that offenders often keep a cache of souvenir images—if located, such images become a permanent record of crime in progress and help identify additional victims, witnesses, and suspects.

6. Address motives. If relevant, review the victim's or witness's motivation for reporting the incident and connect it to observed behavior.

7. Interview and obtain statements from all parties involved, including individuals from other jurisdictions and child protection intervention workers.

   A. Include the victim's statements (if appropriate, considering the victim's age and relationship to potential suspect).

   B. Obtain medical records as appropriate.

8. Determine what occurred by specifying the nature of the criminal event and all overt acts associated with it.

9. If the suspect is on the scene, identify and establish probable cause.

   A. Decide whether to have the suspect voluntarily go to a designated interview area where there may be a more experienced investigator or to make an arrest immediately depending on the circumstances.

   B. Evaluate whether it is appropriate to handcuff the suspect in the presence of the victim or the suspect's family, friends, or coworkers.

   C. Consider circumstances that could adversely affect the likelihood of obtaining a confession.

10. Attempt to obtain a confession from the suspect that meets all criteria associated with current laws. A written statement and, if possible, a videotaped statement can be crucial for successful prosecution.

11. Only officers with the appropriate combination of experience and training should use additional resources such as cameras, videos, anatomical dolls, and evidence collection kits.

SUBSEQUENT INVESTIGATIVE PROCESS
PREPARATION
— Multidisciplinary teams specializing in sexual assault and exploitation should be established to anticipate the victim's needs and conduct a proper and effective investigation.

— Team members include law enforcement officers, social workers, prosecutors, medical practitioners, and counselors.

CHARACTER TRAITS OF INVESTIGATORS

— Authoritative presence paired with calmness

— Extroverted personality, reflected by ability to communicate and show a basic fondness for people

— Professional appearance and sense of being capable (helps suspect perceive investigator as a trustworthy and competent problem solver)

— Accepting and social personality (engenders trust)

— Understands the difference between *guilt* (internally based feeling involving a suspect's conscience) and *shame* (externally based feeling reflecting worry that others will find out about the crime)

1. If the suspect feels more shame than guilt, the likelihood of obtaining a confession decreases.

2. To elicit confession, attempt to minimize a suspect's feeling of shame and accentuate feelings of guilt.

— Able to recognize and address the rationalization process

1. Rationalization is the justification of behavior by faulty logic and involves "poor me" thoughts, feelings of hopelessness and anger, isolationism, inappropriate spontaneous decision making, use of recent life events and previous child abuse as explanations, and use of religious background and confessions to a higher power.

2. Suspects may try to avoid taking responsibility for their actions.

INVESTIGATIVE GOALS

— Identify the full scope of the crime, remembering that cases involving child exploitation through the Internet, child pornography, and child sexual abuse often encompass more than one crime scene and more than one victim.

— Collect and properly record all information associated with the investigation.

— Evaluate all collected data for evidentiary value, noting especially any connection between evidence and suspect.

— Consider all appropriate psychological strategies to obtain a confession or secure evidence.

— Establish rapport with suspects.

— Resolve the case using all resources and skills legally available to police.

— Build a perfect case consisting of 3 elements (investigative trifecta):

1. *Physical evidence showing a relationship between the victim and perpetrator.* Evidence collection and preservation are critical and should be assigned to the most proficient member of the team.

2. *Witnesses with firsthand information.*

3. *Confession from the perpetrator.*

PHYSICAL EVIDENCE

— Keep all attempts to establish facts and gather evidence victim-centered.

— Both types of evidence (***mens rea***, or criminal intent, and ***actus reus***, or criminal act) must be proved in court.

— The most significant sources of evidence are the crime scene and the bodies of the victim and offender.

1. The crime scene expert visits the scene, victim, and offender to identify, locate, and handle evidence.

2. Modern equipment and tools facilitate collection, preservation, photographing, and storing such evidence.

— Examine all material evidence and/or physical signs and psychological symptoms that might connect abuse with the suspect, indicate the way the victim was abused or trafficked, or indicate the means by which abuse or trafficking occurred.

— Evidence includes fibers, written notes, recordings, photographs, traces of body fluids, head or pubic hairs, skin tissue, fingerprints, shoeprints, etc. **Table 8-1** gives further examples.

— The purpose of evidence collection is to substantiate the victim's testimony as well as explain any physical or psychological effects the victim suffered.

— Suggestions for handling a suspect:

1. Use only lawful methods.

2. Control the suspect's access to the victim.

3. If the suspect is arrested immediately, preserve all evidence on the body and clothing.

4. In cases of sexual assault, immediately take the suspect to the hospital for a medical examination.

5. Take photographs of all visible bodily injuries or bruises.

6. Ensure that the suspect does not attempt to destroy or alter evidence or attempt suicide.

Table 8-1. Examples of Evidence

— Souvenirs, including photographs, videos, electronic images, clothing, catalogs, magazines, and all images depicting children, even if not sexual in nature

— Sex toys

— Bindings and sadomasochistic paraphernalia

— Suspect's unwashed clothing and bed linens

— Suspect's DNA

— Suspect's fingerprints

— Cell phone and home phone records

— Computer hard drives, floppy disks, CDs, and DVDs

— Items obtained from search of suspect's employment site (including items from lockers, vehicles, desks, and computers)

— Address books, general and credit card receipts, and cash withdraw and bank records

7. Never interview the suspect until all background information and the facts of the case are obtained.

8. Verify all information gained from the suspect.

9. Arrange for audio and video recordings of the interview.

THE INTERVIEW PROCESS

The Victim

— Be sensitive to the victim who decides to report an assault. Asking the victim for a detailed description of what the offender did and said causes the victim to relive the experience.

— Encourage the victim to have a supportive friend, relative, or counselor present when making the report.

— Be aware of any physical or psychosocial problems the victim has before beginning the interview, and ensure that the victim does not reexperience victimization during the interview.

— Conduct the interview in a comfortable environment where the victim feels safe and secure.

— Wear plain clothes instead of a uniform.

— Ensure the interview lasts no longer than 1 hour at a time.

— Ask open-ended questions and allow the victim time to respond fully.

— Do not change interviewers in the middle of an interview.

— With children:

1. Reinforce behaviors positively.

2. Give appropriate and consistent feedback.

3. Help them verbalize their feelings.

4. Reassure them that they will not be blamed.

5. Victims of pornography production may deny they are depicted in pictures or videos found at the scene or through covert investigations. This is a defense mechanism, and victims will often require more time before they are ready to acknowledge this additional aspect of harm.

6. Victims of prostitution may state that they are not underage and may have been provided with false identification by pimps or offenders. Careful evaluation in a safe and secure location is necessary to obtain the most reliable information.

7. Internationally trafficked victims often have an immense fear of police officers. Obtaining the assistance of an outreach program with people who speak the primary language of the victims is very important to obtain cooperation.

The Suspect

— Based on the evidence, develop a theme, which is a scenario or rationalization used to help the suspect make an admission. This theme ideally minimizes the action of the suspect in the attempt to obtain a confession.

— To develop a theme, be aware of the suspect's frame of mind.

1. Although sexual offender profiles vary, they are usually linked to victimology, motive, and behavior.

    A. Victimology involves detailed assessment of what caused the person to become a victim and how the person was victimized.

    B. Offender's personality and behavior reflect one another.

2. Sexual offenders are more likely to answer key questions if they are presented in way that allows rationalization (see also Chapter 2, Victims and Offenders).

— Evaluate:

1. Previous arrest record

2. Work experience (especially computer expertise in Internet cases)

3. Family background

4. History of childhood sexual abuse

5. History of process addictive behavior, substance addictive behavior, or both

6. Current and past residences

7. Education

8. Social affiliations

9. Experience with pornography, voyeurism, and other paraphilia

10. Victim preference

11. Victim selection and approach

12. Grooming techniques

13. Whether professional help has ever been sought

14. Opinions regarding issues of sexual contact with children and teenagers

— Interviewing tips are listed in **Table 8-2**.

Table 8-2. Interviewing Tips

— Learn as much as possible about the suspect before beginning the interview.

— Attempt to detail the suspect's recent activities, including where the suspect was at the time of the crime and any significant triggers, events, or stressors that the suspect may have experienced recently.

— Obtain background information by interviewing the suspect's associates, family, and friends; then develop an interview strategy.

— Use a standard set of questions to ensure uniformity.

— Schedule the interview or interrogation session so it will not be interrupted.

— Interview the suspect in the police office or a neutral site—never in the suspect's environment.

— Begin by establishing rapport through conversation and nonthreatening, open-ended questions.

— Observe (and possibly have an additional observer) and record in detail the suspect's nonverbal behavior while building rapport.

— When a suspect is deemed responsible for a crime, confront the suspect with the conclusion and utilize themes to elicit a confession or admission of guilt.

— During a confrontation, remain empathetic to the suspect; avoid any condescending or judgmental attitude.

— Other items to remember when interviewing:

1. The power of the police in the interview process is great and can have significant ramifications for the suspect, including loss of freedom, loss of substantial finances, separation from mainstream society, and possibly legal execution.

2. Why offenders may try to deceive an investigator:

   A. Offenders may fear prosecution, termination from a job, embarrassment, restitution, punishment, loss of loving relationships, or may fear for their physical safety.

   B. Offenders may not want to risk losing their profits, especially those offenders involved in pornography.

   C. By understanding the reasons for being deceitful, the investigator can tailor interview questions and evaluate the suspect's reasoning.

3. All statements are relevant. Refusal to make statements or lack of statements is also relevant.

4. Approach each case individually.

5. When multiple theories exist, the most straightforward one is the most likely to be true.

WHEN INVESTIGATIONS FAIL

— Factors that lead to a failed criminal investigation:

1. Tunnel vision or failure to see the big picture

2. Excessive reliance on past experiences

3. Personal interpretation rather than factual analysis of evidence

4. False identification of and false confessions from a suspect

5. Preconceived prejudices based on personal value systems and past conditioning

6. Excessive reliance on intuition, a powerful and emotional force rarely based in fact and prone to error

7. Inability to use logical reasoning and overcome emotions, often

because the physical and psychological trauma of a young victim can be unnerving, making it difficult to suppress emotions

8. Failure to accept external review of case by disinterested parties

INVESTIGATIVE AGENCIES

US POSTAL INSPECTION SERVICE

— Postal inspectors are federal law enforcement officers who carry firearms, make arrests, execute federal search warrants, and serve subpoenas.

— Inspectors:

1. Work closely with US attorneys, other law enforcement agencies, and local prosecutors to investigate cases and prepare them for court.

2. Have specific responsibility for investigating the mailing of obscene matter.

3. Are specially trained to conduct child exploitation investigations and are assigned to each of the US Postal Inspection Service's (USPIS) field divisions nationwide.

4. Use undercover operations to flush out mail-order child pornography dealers; hundreds of offenders are arrested and convicted under new federal laws, such as the Federal Child Protection Act of 1984.

EXPLOITED CHILD UNIT

— The Exploited Child Unit (ECU) exists within the National Center for Missing & Exploited Children (NCMEC) and is designed to better safeguard children from sexual exploitation.

— It serves as a resource center for the public, parents, law enforcement, and others on issues of CSE.

— It performs 3 main services:

1. *CyberTipline.* An online mechanism for the public to report incidences of CSE (NCMEC, 2003). Reports are processed and

leads disseminated to federal, state, local, and international law enforcement agencies for further investigation. It reports possession, manufacturing, and distribution of child pornography; online enticement of children for sexual acts; child prostitution; child sex tourism; extrafamilial child sexual molestation; and the sending of unsolicited obscene material to a child. Most cases are connected to the Internet, though non–Internet-related cases are also handled.

2. *Child Victim Identification Project.* Leading resource on identifying children depicted in child pornography images. Its goals are to identify child victims and assist law enforcement agencies and prosecutors in enhancing prosecutions of federal, state, and local cases of child pornography and CSE. The most beneficial resource of the project is a broad knowledge base of child victims who have been identified by law enforcement in previous investigations. This base consists of:

   A. The Child Recognition & Identification System, a computer application developed by NCMEC to scan and select image files containing such child victims. It identifies images based on the MD5 hash values (a mathematical algorithm) to verify that one file matches another exactly. After images are analyzed, a Child Identification Report is generated, specifying exact file names and contact information for the specific police officer who interviewed the child.

   B. The Child Pornography Evidence Guide, which assists law enforcement in becoming familiar with child pornography series containing identified children. It contains child pornography series name(s), comprehensive series description (sexual activity, background, physical descriptions), series identifiers (distinct items, clothing, tattoos), and partial file names. The project is continually being revised to reflect newest series. See Chapter 9, Investigating Child Pornography, for more information on methods of identifying children.

3. *Exploited Child Unit Technical Assistance Services.* Experts assist in any child exploitation case (**Table 8-3**).

Table 8-3. Technical Assistance Services Available From the Exploited Child Unit Internet Searches

ECU analysts have extensive training in data collection using the Internet. Analysts use Internet resources to gather information on Web sites, e-mail addresses, newsgroup postings, and suspect locations as well as other important pieces of information relevant to the case. Many times the ECU analyst is able to provide information to the requesting agency with a detailed list of the suspect's Internet activities.

PUBLIC RECORD DATABASE SEARCHES

The ECU has access to several public record databases that may yield critical information on suspects such as Social Security and/or drivers' license numbers, past criminal history, and recent addresses.

CYBERTIPLINE HISTORICAL SEARCHES

As of July 2003, there were more than 135 000 reports in the CyberTipline and technical assistance databases, and they continue to grow by more than 1000 reports a week. ECU analysts can search these databases for previous reports related to current investigations using various criteria such as suspect names, e-mail addresses, Web addresses, and even text phrases.

TECHNICAL EXPERTISE

The computer skills and knowledge of the ECU analysts are continually developing and expanding as the Internet continues to evolve. Analysts have a pool of expert knowledge on the various programs, software, and technology used on the Internet today in forums such as peer-to-peer networks, the World Wide Web, e-mail applications, Internet Relay Chat, and File Transfer Protocol.

LAW ENFORCEMENT CONTACTS

CyberTipline leads are received from all over the world; therefore, the ECU is continually establishing new contacts with domestic and international law enforcement agencies that specialize in child exploitation cases. These contacts may be beneficial for multijurisdictional and multinational cases.

(continued)

Table 8-3. *(continued)*

INTERNET SERVICE PROVIDER (ISP) CONTACTS

Since 1999, ISPs have been required to report child pornography to the CyberTipline per 42 USC § 13032(B)(1). ISPs are able to provide law enforcement with evidence, subscriber information, and user history. The ECU has an extensive list of ISP contact names, telephone numbers, and e-mail addresses to assist law enforcement in accessing information.

PUBLICATIONS

The NCMEC has numerous publications available on Internet safety and preventing, understanding, and investigating child sexual exploitation. Copies of these publications are available online at http://www.missingkids.com or may be obtained by calling 1-800-843-5678.

TRAINING

The NCMEC, in conjunction with various partners, offers numerous courses several times a year all around the nation to train professionals on investigating and preventing child exploitation. The NCMEC Legal Resource Division offers training in specialized skills needed by prosecutors, judges, and law enforcement officers on how to adjudicate these cases successfully. In addition, it also provides technical assistance in the investigation and prosecution of violent crimes against children.

LAW ENFORCEMENT PARTNERSHIPS
—The NCMEC is not an investigative agency, but several federal agencies are represented at its headquarters in Virginia.

—The Federal Bureau of Investigation, Bureau of Immigration and Customs Enforcement, USPIS, US Secret Service, and Bureau of Alcohol, Tobacco and Firearms have personnel assigned to work at NCMEC's headquarters, serve as liaisons to their respective agencies, and assist NCMEC's staff with case analysis and investigative support.

REFERENCE
National Center for Missing & Exploited Children. The Cyber-Tipline. 2003. Available at: http://www.cybertipline.com. Accessed September 19, 2003.

Chapter 9

INVESTIGATING CHILD PORNOGRAPHY

Sharon W. Cooper, MD, FAAP
Terry Jones, BA (Hons), PGCE

MEDICAL ANALYSIS IN PORNOGRAPHY

See also Chapter 7, Medical Issues.

— Medical analysis of child pornography is not an absolute requirement because most child sexual abuse images clearly depict children. Medical analysis is most often sought when the ages of subjects in pornographic images are questionable.

— Medical analysis is used to assess a victim's age, which is then used to determine whether the evidence meets the criteria of the law regarding child pornography.

— It may identify the victim in the image and help locate that victim.

— Medical analysis can yield information about a collector's specific fetish or behavioral pattern.

— It can assess the images produced by the collector to find evidence that may be used in further investigation.

— Medical analysis creates a document of what the sexual abuse images show. The COPINE stages can be used to categorize the acts and can alleviate the need for visualization of images in court proceedings when there is judicial aversion (see **Table 3-1**).

VICTIM IDENTIFICATION ANALYSIS

— A significant amount of child pornography is made in the home and by a child's family members; carefully question the child and friends because delayed disclosure is common.

— When viewing images, include all of the people shown, noting and commenting on children in the background.

— False images of child abuse (pseudo images) exist in relatively low numbers.

1. These images are created by manually or digitally replacing heads on adult pornographic images with those of children.

2. Alternatively, adult features can be altered to present a more childlike body image.

— Some limited examples of computer-generated pseudo images are also available.

— The victim identification process is designed to determine who the children are, where they are, when an image was created, whether children have been found, and who should investigate the crime.

GENDER

— Generally, determining the gender of a child depicted in a sexual abuse image is not difficult.

1. Only state what is visible in the image.

2. If the child's body has evidence of waist definition (indicative of the deposition of fat typically found in adolescent females) or if the shoulder-to-hip ratio is 1.35 or greater (indicative of maturation often seen in older adolescent males), make a tentative determination of gender.

3. Using hair length to decide a child's gender is unreliable.

4. When an image is of a young child, clear designation of gender is often difficult to discern unless the genitals are revealed.

5. When pornographic images include only a child's head (usually in profile) performing fellatio on a man, do not speculate about the child's gender. However, the relative size of the child's head next to an erect penis is usually enough information to determine whether the image is actually that of a child.

6.   Because videotape pornography often shows large groups of children, analysis requires the ability to slow the tape down and evaluate each subject completely. Even if most of the children seem to be of 1 gender, cross-dressing is sometimes depicted, so each child must be analyzed.

ETHNICITY

— Ethnic origin (ancestry) is especially relevant to victim identification.

1.   Sexually abused and exploited children are usually photographed in their country of origin.

2.   If they are transported to another country, human trafficking and prostitution may be taking place and involve a large-scale, commercial, organized crime operation.

3.   Increase the index of suspicion if an ethnic business is the site of pornography production.

4.   Meta-analysis of the background environment of Internet images is key in victim identification.

— For clinical indications to determine ethnicity, refer to Chapter 7, Medical Issues.

— **Table 9-1** lists the general characteristics of the major ethnic groups.

— Facial features of children of African descent vary tremendously based on multiethnic background.

1.   African American children show a prevalence of racial mixing.

2.   Children from certain African countries have an appearance consistent with their specific nation of origin.

3.   Children of African descent are less often posted pornographically and are not often seen in multiple series of child pornography.

— Other clues that help determine a child's ethnicity include:

1.   Video titles and Internet Web site banners. They are often accurate regarding subject matter of the associated images.

Table 9-1. General Facial Characteristics of Major Ethnic Groups

EUROPEAN ANCESTRY

— Minimal projection.

— Relative small zygomatic arches, which give face relatively narrow appearance across midface and narrow nasal appearance.

— Typically receding lower eye border.

— Possible presence of hypertelorism or hypotelorism (increased or decreased distance between eyes, respectively, though this is often genetic instead of an ancestry trait).

HISPANIC ANCESTRY

— Dark hair.

— Almond-shaped eyes.

— Somewhat darker complexion than those of European descent, with a subjectively more olive tone; those of direct Spanish descent still have European characteristics.

ASIAN ANCESTRY

— Characteristic body habitus (shorter stature, small features in girls).

— Dark hair.

— Almond-shaped, upward slanting eyes.

— Upper and lower eyelids appear fuller than those of other races; orbital fat projects further both anteriorly and superiorly to the inferior border of the tarsus (Carter et al, 1998).

— Skin pigment less uniform than other ethnic groups because children have darker pigment associated with greater sun exposure or may be wearing makeup to appear extremely fair (common in some Asian countries).

— Children from some parts of Eurasia may be as hyperpigmented as children of African descent.

AFRICAN ANCESTRY

— Skin tone and complexion show various degrees of pigmentation.

— Dark hair.

— Round eyes.

— Relatively broad nasal bridge.

— Projection of alveolar ridge.

— Rarely crowded dentition, which is often seen in European children.

2. Stereotypical settings of the country of origin, such as Hispanic children in exotic, tropical environments or the use of known European sites.

3. Background scenes that provide clues to country in which pornography production occurs. Once the country of origin is determined for some pornographic pictures, some victims can be successfully located. This is particularly true in a room that constitutes a crime scene from a law enforcement standpoint.

AGE

— Toddler pornography

1. Child pornography collections often show infants, toddlers (aged 12 to 36 months), or preschool-aged children (37 to 60 months).

2. Different developmental stages may provide an indication of the degree of maturation present in younger children.

3. If viewing videotapes or Internet video clips of sexual abuse images, observe a child's gross motor skills to help identify developmental level (**Table 9-2**).

4. Toddler photography may show a nude male child bending over and looking through his legs. This highlights the presence of the anus and testes, since the penis is too small to be seen in much detail. The ability to stand this way begins to appear at age 14.5 to 15.5 months.

5. Sadistic toddler abuse: Toddler pornography is increasingly associated with vaginal, anal, or oral penetration. The victim may wear additional "props" such as a spiked dog collar around the neck, blindfold over the eyes, gag in the mouth, or rope tied around the ankles or wrists.

— Dental maturation

1. Eruption and shedding of teeth are helpful parameters for analyzing images of young children.

2. Tooth eruption occurs at a fairly predictable rate in infants and toddlers.

Table 9-2. Stages of Development of Gross Motor Skills in Toddlers

— *Walking independently.* Toddler is probably between 11.5 and 13.5 months old and usually younger than 15 months old, which is the upper limit for normal development. (Note: African American children tend to walk 2 to 4 months earlier than other children.)

— *Walking backward when pulling an object (eg, a toy).* Toddler is probably between 12.5 and 21 months old.

— *Walking with high-guard or mid-guard stance with wide-based foot placement.* Toddler is probably between 13 and 15 months old.

— *Standing and looking through legs.* Toddler is probably older than 14.5 to 15.5 months.

— *Walking facing forward and pulling an object behind the body with one hand.* Toddler is probably between 15 and 18 months old.

— *Carrying a large object while walking.* Toddler is probably between 17 and 18.5 months old.

— *Squatting during play.* Toddler is probably older than 20 to 21 months.

---

3. **Table 9-3** lists the chronology of human dentition for primary and secondary teeth.

4. Tooth shedding can be altered by poor nutrition, poverty, and dental caries.

— Physical sexual maturation

1. Norms of sexual maturation are based on actual physical examinations of children whose ages are known. When only pictures are available, it is only possible to determine approximate height ratios, body habitus, dentition, muscular development, dysmorphia, and physical sexual maturation.

2. Tanner stages: See **Figures 9-1** through **9-3** (Marshall & Tanner, 1969, 1970; Tanner, 1962).

3. Age ranges cited in original Tanner research are unsuitable for child pornography analysis. They were devised for the purpose of

clinical medical investigation rather than forensic analysis aimed at victim assessment and possible identification (Marshall & Tanner, 1986).

4. More recent sexual maturation ratings with correlative ages provide an enhanced background for the analysis of sexual abuse images.

5. Observe children's developmental cues and compare observations with the most recent data available regarding median age of each stage of development.

6. Use the age of entry into a given stage of pubertal development to determine children's greatest degree of potential immaturity.

7. Pubic hair distribution is the most obvious and reliable gauge of sexual maturation in child pornography. In girls, breast development usually precedes the onset of pubic hair growth by a few months. When a significant discrepancy is noted, choose the age of the more advanced sexual maturation rating value.

8. Accepted sequence of puberty changes in girls—breast development, pubic hair, axillary hair, menses. Premature breast development (thelarche) and premature pubarche require endocrinologic evaluation, but these conditions are rare and should not be considered when assessing child pornography.

9. The cycle of puberty requires 5 to 6 years for completion (Grumbach & Styne, 1998). If the photographed child has not attained complete adult sexual maturation, the child is most likely younger than 18 years.

10. Delayed or early sexual maturation may occur in persons with rare genetic conditions (see Chapter 7, Medical Issues).

EVIDENCE
PROPER HANDLING
See **Table 9-4**.

Eliminate the Risk of Possible Courtroom Confusion or Exclusion of Evidence

Table 9-3. Chronology of Human Dentition for Primary (Deciduous) and Secondary (Permanent) Teeth

PRIMARY TEETH	CALCIFICATION		AGE AT ERUPTION		AGE AT SHEDDING	
	BEGINS AT	COMPLETES AT	MAXILLARY	MANDIBULAR	MAXILLARY	MANDIBULAR
Central incisors	5th fetal month	18-24 months	6-8 months	5-7 months	7-8 years	6-7 years
Lateral incisors	5th fetal month	18-24 months	8-11 months	7-10 months	8-9 months	7-8 months
Cuspids (canines)	6th fetal month	30-36 months	16-20 months	16-20 months	11-12 years	9-11 years
First molars	5th fetal month	24-30 months	10-16 months	10-16 months	10-11 years	10-12 years
Second molars	6th fetal month	36 months	20-30 months	20-30 months	10-12 years	11-13 years

SECONDARY TEETH	BEGINS AT	COMPLETES AT	MAXILLARY	MANDIBULAR		
Central incisors	3-4 months	9-10 years	7-8 years	6-7 years		
Lateral incisors	Maxillary, 10-12 months; Mandibular, 3-4 months	10-11 years	8-9 years	7-8 years		
Cuspids (canines)	4-5 months	12-15 years	11-12 years	9-11 years		

First premolars (bicuspids)	18-21 months	12-13 years	10-11 years	10-12 years
Second molars (bicuspids)	24-30 months	12-14 years	10-12 years	11-13 years
First molars	Birth	9-10 years	6-7 years	6-7 years
Second molars	30-36 months	14-16 years	12-13 years	12-13 years
Third molars	Maxillary, 7-9 years; Mandibular, 8-10 years	18-25 years	17-22 years	17-22 years

Reprinted with permission from Behrman & Kliegman, 2000.

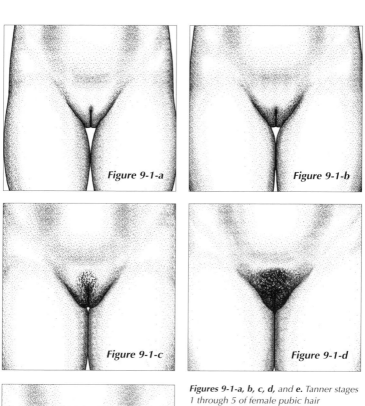

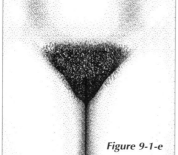

Figures 9-1-a, b, c, d, and *e.* Tanner stages 1 through 5 of female pubic hair development.

Figures 9-2-a, b, c, d, and *e.* Tanner stages 1 through 5 of female breast development.

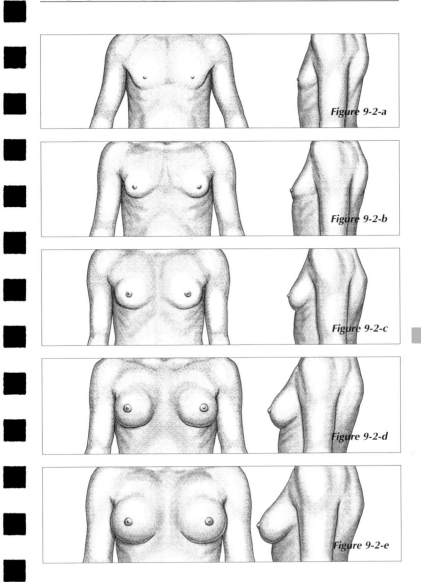

Figure 9-2-a

Figure 9-2-b

Figure 9-2-c

Figure 9-2-d

Figure 9-2-e

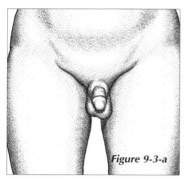

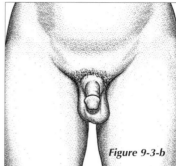

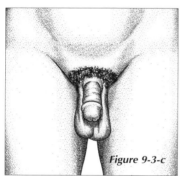

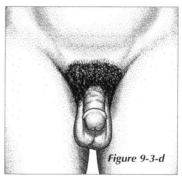

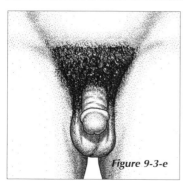

Figures 9-3-a, b, c, d, and **e.** Tanner stages 1 through 5 of male pubic hair and genitalia development.

Table 9-4. Recommendations for the Proper Handling of Child Pornography Evidence

— Properly label all images if there are not file names already assigned.

— Indicate the investigation case number and computer-based image file number for each image.

— Be able to verify that the images were secured while in the possession of the medical expert.

— Be able to verify that the evaluation of the images pertains specifically to the case in question and that there is no chance that images from another case were included during the expert evaluation.

— Be extremely sensitive and strive to ensure that the child victim is not further exploited by the court proceedings.

— Verify that the images have been secured while in the investigator's possession to ensure that they have had no opportunity to mix with images of other cases.

— In all instances, ensure that the images reviewed are for the specific case and none belong to another case.

Eliminate the Risk of Further Exploitation of the Victim
— Be sensitive to the needs of the child.

— Respect the privacy of the victim even if the victim's identity remains unknown.

— This creates a standard for the entire multidisciplinary team as well as the court with respect to the need to protect the victim.

RECEIPT OF EVIDENCE
— Use the original source to avoid further reproduction of images. This is especially pertinent if images were found on a computer or another electronic means of storage.

— If the images are published in magazines or stored as photographs in an album, perform an on-site review to avoid further exploitation of the children in the images.

— When images are stored as videos, a review usually requires personal access to the video. Clips may be inserted into videos of benign content, and finding and analyzing multiple images and subjects to be analyzed may take a significant amount of time.

Receipt of Photographs and Videos
— If time or distance prevents traveling to review images, have evidence delivered in the "badge-to-badge" method.

1.   This method involves coordination between law enforcement agencies.

2.   The Federal Bureau of Investigation, US Customs and Border Protection, Department of Homeland Security, and US Postal Inspection Service frequently handle this form of contraband and are well versed in the appropriate manner of ensuring chain of custody is maintained in the United States.

3.   The International Criminal Police Organization (Interpol and its affiliates) facilitates these issues outside of the United States.

— Document when and from whom the evidence is received (certified mail, hand-delivered, commercial carrier) and include the information in the case file.

— Safekeeping:

1.   Keep child pornography in a secure place during analysis so there is no risk of legal challenge that images were altered.

2.   Track the return of evidence so clear documentation exists.

3.   Do not transmit analyses of such cases by electronic mail. Send an original document with a personal signature and provide the tracking of the report. This procedure ensures that discovery can be provided in a timely fashion.

Receipt of Computer-Based Evidence
— If copies of images were made available for review, evidence should be provided on CD-ROM so that the medical analysis of individual images can be conducted and images enlarged if needed.

— Review evidence in a way that avoids copying images onto a computer hard drive, since storage of such contraband could constitute a violation of existing laws.

— Sometimes copies of images are provided as printouts.

1. Copies should be made in color and larger than a typical ***thumbnail*** (file format used by imaging software, usually with a file extension of ".thn").

2. Enlarged copies are preferred to ease analysis.

3. If enlarged copies are not available, access to magnification capabilities may be necessary.

4. If possible, include in the documentation of computer-based images the complete file name of each image. Include the investigation case number, the total number of images considered to have met the criteria for child pornography, and the total number of images provided for medical analysis. Investigative agencies might only submit a percentage of the total number of images because they tend to select images that appear most like children.

— The burden of proof is on investigators to ensure that at least 1 image in a collection is of a known victim (*Ashcroft v Free Speech Coalition*, 2002).

1. Requiring identification of at least 1 victim provides a greater motivation to identify children who have been sexually abused in this manner.

2. Although a medical analyst may provide information for the court, at least 1 child must already have been identified for the case to proceed.

The Prosecutorial Remedies and Other Tools to end the Exploitation of Children Today (PROTECT) Act
— Defines child pornography images as those that, to an ordinary observer, are of an actual minor.

— Allows the accused to escape prosecution if they can prove the images were not produced using real children.

— The medical analyst may be asked whether digital modification of the images (a process known as morphing) exists.

1. Determination requires advanced computer skills and ability, and so forensic computer experts who have access to significant image magnification tools and the ability to analyze pixel definition, color variations, and other factors should conduct the analysis.

2. Forensic medical analysis is specifically for determining image content, not image quality. As a result, it is unwise for medical analysts to try to determine whether an image was morphed unless they have received advanced training in computer forensic analysis or had access to a prior report addressing this issue at the time of medical analysis.

3. When morphing is obvious, it often includes the image of a well-known person's face being placed on the body image of someone else. A medical analyst can comment on such images; however, morphed images are not necessary for analysis. The medical analyst can use such an image in a trial as a demonstrative aid to ensure that the analysis is serious and does not include nonsensical images.

VIDEOTAPE EVIDENCE

— When reviewing videotaped evidence, use a videotape player able to either freeze screens or display frames at a rate sufficiently slow to afford careful visualization of the images.

— Because child pornography may be inserted into videos of other subjects, view the entire videotape.

— The videotape identification number may be an investigation case file number.

— Identify the title of the videotape because it usually suggests the juvenile nature of content.

— Information can lend support to the intent of the offender to collect contraband that is child pornography as opposed to a claim of ignorance about the videotape's subject matter.

Inserted Pornographic Vignettes
— Crime scene investigations have found pornographic clips within children's cartoon videos as well as in the middle of action movies.

— Determine the amount of time that pornography is displayed via this form of media.

— Give a brief description of the vignette to permit the triers of fact the opportunity to be familiar with the content without viewing the entire videotape.

— The medical analyst's description of the content is relevant because a judge may not allow the actual contraband to be viewed in the courtroom due to the video's potentially prejudicial nature. During a trial, an analyst's report allows the jury or judge the opportunity to understand the explicit nature of the content and the degree of exploitation evident.

Unusual Angles Shown in the Video
— Discern whether any identifying aspects of images shown at unusual angles indicate the presence of a child seen previously in the video.

— Ensure with a reasonable certainty that these unusual views are of the original child.

— Since these views are often sexually explicit, they can portray hair distribution on both the child's and the perpetrator's bodies. The absence of axillary hair or the pubic hair distribution can help determine the child's sexual maturity.

Partial Image of a Perpetrator
— If there is an identified suspect in the case, limit analysis to frames of videotape that confirm the suspect's identity.

— Suspect evaluation may include photos of the suspect's body, and these photos may be used for comparison.

— If hands are visible in suspect detainment photographs, details (fingernails, venous pattern on dorsum of hand, identifying body marks) may be analyzed to determine whether the suspect's features are consistent with those of the person shown in the videotape.

— Supportive evidence of the suspect's role in the production of child pornography is also possible.

Multiple Subjects in a Video
— Videotapes of child pornography may be commercially available and frequently include multiple child and teenaged subjects. Analysis of this evidence is especially time consuming because 1 tape, which is often a compilation of several short vignettes, may have 40 or more subjects.

— These tapes often do not have an audio background; they are commonly filmed in Europe, South America, or Central America.

— Most show teenaged subjects initially clothed, but as the video continues, they often become naked and participate in sexual activity.

— The "actors" in these videotapes usually are believed to be homeless children and/or young people who have been coerced into juvenile prostitution.

— Analysis of such a video:

1. Be careful to describe each child or young person separately.

2. One method of labeling the young subjects is according to the sequence of their appearance in the video.

3. Provide a brief, body-identifying description (eg, race and hair color) that adequately indicates to another observer which young person is being analyzed.

4. **Figure 9-4** illustrates a model worksheet for identifying subjects according to order of appearance in a video.

   A. First, each subject is assigned a letter according to the subject's appearance in the video.

   B. A brief description of the subject may be provided in an adjoining column.

Multiple Victim Child Pornography Analysis Sheet

VIDEO & TITLE:_____

Vignette
#1_____
_____

Subjects		PH	G	B	Other Findings	Meets Criteria
A						
B						
C						
D						
E						
F						
G						
H						
I						
J						

Vignette
#2_____
_____

Subjects		PH	G	B	Other Findings	Meets Criteria
A						
B						
C						
D						
E						
F						
G						
H						
I						
J						

Figurre 9-4. *A worksheet like this can be helpful to organize the descriptions of multiple subjects in one video.*

    C. Sexual maturation ratings can be assigned, and other details (eg, presence of axillary hair, muscle development, head-to-body ratio) can be included.

    D. A final column exists for the examiner's determination of whether the subject's appearance is consistent with that of a youth younger than 18 years or a child younger than 12 years.

    E. This final column also allows space to designate whether the images meet the definition of child erotica in accordance with US laws.

— Images defined as erotica in the United States may not meet another country's legal criteria for child pornography.

Information About Child Seduction
— Modus operandi may be depicted.

— Pornography may provide a blueprint for action to a sex offender.

Incest Shown on a Videotape
— These tapes often include a sound track.

— Content usually supports the observation that most sexual abuse of children occurs in a familiar setting and by a family member, friend, or acquaintance.

PHOTOGRAPHS AND PUBLISHED MATERIALS AS EVIDENCE
— Carefully document the evidence number to avoid confusion.

— If photographs for review have not been labeled by law enforcement officials or are given to the reviewer as a group or collection and labeled only by the date of the investigation, assign a label to each image.

1.   Labels should preferably describe the content to minimize problems when discussing specific photographs.

2.   Another way to define the images is to request that investigators assign a specific name or number to each picture.

3.   *Example*: A case file includes a homemade photo album with combinations of child erotica and child pornography images.

Initially, the reviewer comments on the entire file and the total number of pictures in the album. Further analysis determines which images constitute child pornography, child erotica, etc. The album is then cited as part of the contraband for that case.

Written Child Pornography

— Collections of written pornography about adults and children may be found on a suspect's hard drive or at the scene.

— This form of pornography is generally protected by the First Amendment of the US Constitution.

— The presence of such stories in child sexual exploitation cases serves the following purposes:

1.   Provides sex offender with a rationalization for such behavior

2.   Allows the sex offender to fantasize about being seduced by a young child and trying to resist this seduction

3.   May memorialize an actual event in the form of fiction for some offenders

— The significance of finding written child pornography in a suspect's possession is similar to that of finding child erotica: Neither form is illegal, but both imply a preferential interest in sex with children.

— Other information often found with written child pornography:

1.   Tables of international ages of sexual consent, which provide the collector with more information supporting child sexual tourism or sexual fantasy

2.   Information about various groups that advocate sex with children

Child Erotica Images

— Differentiate child pornography from child erotica.

1.   *Child pornography.* Depicts child sexual abuse and constitutes a crime scene.

2.   *Child erotica.* Does not depict sexual abuse but may be highly suggestive and ultimately serve the purpose of a fantasy source for

a collector. May include images taken from store catalogs for children's clothing.

3. *Internet child erotica.* Pictures of children that do not meet the standard for sexual abuse images but are included in a collection of images that contain child pornography.

— Erotica may be found on a suspect's computer and included in an analysis.

ROLE OF POSTAL INSPECTORS
See Chapter 8, Principles of Investigation.

REFERENCES

Ashcroft v Free Speech Coalition, 535 US 234 (9th Cir 2002).

Behrman RE, Kleigman RM, Jenson HB, eds. *Nelson's Textbook of Pediatrics.* 16th ed. Philadelphia, Pa: WB Saunders Company; 2000.

Carter SR, Seiff S, Grant PE, Vigneron DB. The Asian lower eyelid: a comparative anatomic study using high-resolution magnetic resonance imaging. *Ophthal Plas Reconstr Surg.* 1998;14(4):227-234.

Grumbach MM, Styne DM. Puberty: ontogeny, neuroendocrinology, physiology, and disorders. In: Wilson JD, Foster DW, Kronenberg HM, Larsen PR, eds. *Williams Textbook of Endocrinology.* 9th ed. Philadelphia, Pa: WB Saunders; 1998:1509-1625.

Marshall W, Tanner JM. Puberty. In: Falkner F, Tanner JM, eds. *Postnatal Growth: Neurobiology.* 2nd ed. New York, NY: Plenum Press; 1986:171-209. *Human Growth: A Comprehensive Treatise*; vol 2.

Marshall W, Tanner JM. Variations in the pattern of pubertal changes in girls. *Arch Dis Child.* 1969;44:291-303.

Marshall W, Tanner JM. Variation in the pattern or pubertal changes in boys. *Arch Dis Child.* 1970;45:13-23.

Tanner JM. *Growth at Adolescence.* 2nd ed. Springfield, Ill: Charles C Thomas; 1962.

Chapter 10

Investigating the Prostitution of Children

Susan S. Kreston, JD, LLM

— The investigation of prostituted children requires specialized staff members (multidisciplinary team comprising investigators, prosecutors, victim advocates, social workers, and other allied professionals) trained for child exploitation cases.

— Smaller jurisdictions can designate 1 officer who has expertise and a commitment to working in this field (Vieth, 1998).

Gathering Evidence

— All of the investigative techniques used in other felony investigations are applicable to these cases, but the focus is on suspect interrogation.

— The information gathered at this stage may prove critical at the charging phase and during the trial itself.

— Investigators need training in the best practices for interviewing both intrafamilial and extrafamilial child abusers and exploiters.

— Witness interviews and informants' statements are also important.

— Surveillance of the scene(s) where prostitution takes place (on the street, at escort services, in massage parlors, through computer "dating" services, etc) should be undertaken.

— Videotaping of scenes may help bring the jury into the world of the exploited child during the trial.

— Subpoenas and search warrants may be needed to gain information and evidence pertinent to these cases.

INVESTIGATIVE APPROACHES

— Pretext calls, in states where this strategy is legal, may be worth considering; however, careful consideration must be given to the victim's psychological ability to perform this task and to the possibility that the victim may use the opportunity to alert the subject.

— Reverse sting e-mails, in which the investigator takes over an existing e-mail correspondence with the suspect, can be used.

— Sting operations and undercover investigations are also successful, proactive approaches (*United States v Spruill*, 2002).

— **Table 10-1** lists specific questions and issues to address during an investigation.

— See also Chapter 8, Principles of Investigation.

VICTIM INTERVIEWS

— When talking to a victim, do not use the word *pimp* unless the victim does; instead, use whatever name or description the victim uses, such as friend or boyfriend.

— If children refer to themselves as hustlers or escorts, utilize that language accordingly.

— Do not convey a judgmental attitude.

— Children may be noncooperative, sullen, recalcitrant, or emotional.

— Identifying prostituted children can be difficult because many appear older than their age and view police officers as the enemy.

1. Interview these children immediately and record the interview.

2. Videotape the interview if possible.

— Use of a forensic interview specialist is encouraged: They are trained experts in interviewing the victims in these cases, especially teenaged victims.

— Since victims may be cooperating or compliant (Lanning, 2002) and may not actively disclose their abuse, use of a child interview specialist is highly advised.

Table 10-1. Issues to Be Addressed During the Investigation

1. How was the victim recruited? At what age was the victim recruited?

2. What is the name of the pimp and his or her street name(s) or alias(es)?

3. Did the pimp provide instructions to the victim about the way the process worked?

4. Did the pimp receive the money directly, indirectly, or in another manner?

5. Did the pimp use or threaten violence?

6. Did the victim ever receive medical treatment?

7. Can the victim identify any other victims and prostituted adults with whom the victim had contact? If so, what were their street names, aliases, or stage names? Were any of these other victims and/or adults ever arrested? Did any of them show the victim the way the process worked?

8. What mode of prostitution was used (eg, track, services, front companies)?

9. If travel was involved, what mode of transportation was used? Who paid for the transportation? Was it by bus or air carrier? If so, what were the dates?

10. If hotels were used, what were their names and descriptions? Who paid for these hotels?

11. Identify the victim's terms (eg, define "sex") during the forensic interview.

12. Did the victim have sex with the pimp?

13. Did the victim ever become pregnant? If so, what happened to that pregnancy? If the pregnancy was terminated, when, where, and by whom did this occur?

— Prostituted children and youths are almost always victims of intimate partner violence and the dynamics of interviewing in that scenario apply.

— Consider obtaining a medical evaluation because of the associated health problems with prostitution, including physical abuse, substance abuse, mental health problems with trauma, depression or anxiety, and sexually transmitted diseases.

COORDINATION OF EFFORTS

— If the case crosses departmental divisions (vice, juvenile, child abuse), units must coordinate their efforts to obtain the best investigation and assist the child.

— Decisions regarding who will lead the investigation are made on the basis of probable charges and available penalties in each area, personnel and economic resources available in each area, and amount of experience with these cases.

— Priority and importance allotted to these cases should be the same as for any other sex crimes committed against children.

SEARCH AND SEIZURE OF COMPUTER EVIDENCE

Includes address books, biographies, calendars, customer database and/or records, e-mails, notes, letters, false identification, financial asset records, Internet activity logs, medical records, and Web page advertising

DISPOSITION OF SUSPECTS AND VICTIMS

— Individuals who engage in prostitution should be arrested for prostituting a child, molestation, rape, or other factually appropriate child sexual abuse violations. The crimes for which individuals are arrested directly affect amount of bail set before formal charging by the prosecutor's office.

— Children who have been violated should be taken into mandatory protective custody and released into the custody of protective services. Prostituted children are to be treated as victims and not criminals.

REFERENCES

Lanning KV. The compliant and cooperating victim. *APSAC Advisor*. (Special issue) 2002;14(2):4-9.

United States v Spruill, 296 F3d 580 (7th Cir 2002).

Vieth VI. In my neighbor's house: a proposal to address child abuse in rural America. *Hamline Law Rev*. 1998;22:143.

Chapter 11

INVESTIGATING CYBER-ENTICEMENT

Cormac Callanan, BA, MSc
Terry Jones, BA (Hons), PGCE
John Patzakis, Esq
Thomas Rickert, president of INHOPE
Sp Agt Christopher D. Trifiletti

PRINCIPLES OF INVESTIGATION

— Goal is the recovery of evidence and intelligence during the postarrest examination of computers.

1. The information is valuable nationally and internationally to identify other unknown offenders and child victims (Holland, 2003).

2. Identifying the types of images a suspect saves indicates the suspect's interests.

3. The information will be an integral part of the subsequent child protection risk assessment process.

— *Computer forensics* is the discipline dedicated to the collection, analysis, and presentation of computer evidence for judicial purposes.

1. Nearly all child pornography cases involve digital images.

2. Investigators must be familiar with the laws of evidence in their relevant jurisdictions to use proper procedures, tools, and methods to collect and process computer evidence.

— See **Appendix 11-1** for a glossary of Internet terms.

THE INVESTIGATIVE PROCESS

— Involves 3 components: enforcement, training, and education.

— **Table 11-1** depicts the matrix of discovery and investigation of child exploitation on the Internet.

— **Table 11-2** shows how to minimize the chances of an online exploiter victimizing a child.

IDENTIFYING SUSPECTS AND POTENTIAL INTERNET CRIME AREAS

— Obtain information by reading posted material and by monitoring known areas that draw potential abusers.

— Resulting intelligence identifies who posted the information.

— Suspects can be identified from citizen and/or parent complaints.

— Technical and professional sources provide information that helps focus resources on suspects.

— Internet child sexual exploitation (CSE) complaints typically comprise 2 violations:

1. Complaints about child pornography (trader case)

2. Complaints about people attempting to meet children via the Internet for sexual exploitation purposes (traveler case)

— The term *child abuse images* is preferred to *child pornography* in international situations.

INVESTIGATIVE TASK FORCE

PURPOSE AND MEMBERS

— Investigative skills and resources are pooled in the task force concept.

— Task forces:

1. Include members of multiple agencies and jurisdictions.

2. Ensure the best chance of identifying and arresting offenders.

3. Permit sharing of expensive computer and labor resources as well as criminal intelligence.

Table 11-1. Investigators and Complainants

ONLINE INVESTIGATORS

— Federal Bureau of Investigation (FBI)

— Immigration and Customs Enforcement (ICE)

— US Postal Inspection Service (USPIS)

— Internet Crimes Against Children (ICAC) task forces

LAW ENFORCEMENT COMPLAINANTS

— FBI offices and legats

— ICE field offices and attaches

— USPIS field offices

— Police departments

CIVILIAN COMPLAINANTS

— National Center for Missing & Exploited Children (NCMEC)

— Internet service providers (ISPs)

— Child advocates

— Physicians and other healthcare providers

CHILDREN AND FAMILIES

Table 11-2. What Can You Do to Minimize the Chances of an Online Exploiter Victimizing Your Child?

— Communicate with your child about sexual victimization and potential online danger.

— Spend time with your children online. Have them teach you about their favorite online destinations.

— Keep the computer in a common room in the house, not in your child's bedroom. It is much more difficult for a sex offender to communicate with a child when the computer screen is visible to a parent or another member of the household.

(continued)

Table 11-2. *(continued)*

— Use parental controls provided by your ISP and/or blocking software but do not totally rely on them. Although an electronic chat room can be a great place for children to make new friends and discuss various topics of interest, it is also prowled by computer sex offenders. Use of chat rooms, in particular, should be heavily monitored.

— Always maintain access to your child's online account and randomly check his/her e-mail. Be aware that your child could be contacted through the US mail. Be upfront with your child about your access and reasons why.

— Teach your child the responsible use of online resources. There is more to the online experience than chat rooms.

— Find out what computer safeguards are used by your child's school, the public library, and at the homes of your child's friends. These are all places, outside of your normal supervision, where your child could encounter an online predator.

— Understand, even if your child was a willing participant in any form of sexual exploitation, that he/she is not at fault and is the victim. The offender always bears the complete responsibility for his or her actions.

— Instruct your children never to do the following:

— Arrange a face-to-face meeting with someone they met online

— Upload (post) pictures of themselves onto the Internet or online service to people they do not personally know

— Give out identifying information such as their name, home address, school name, or telephone number

— Download pictures from an unknown source as there could be sexually explicit images

— Respond to messages or bulletin board postings that are suggestive, obscene, belligerent, or harassing

— Believe whatever they are told online; it may or may not be true

Adapted from Federal Bureau of Investigation (FBI), 2004.

— Sometimes 1 person performs several roles simultaneously, as with a smaller task force (**Figure 11-1**), but the principal roles are:

1. *Coordinators.* Serve as liaisons between other task force members and law enforcement agencies.

2. *Computer forensics examiners.* Review the equipment and media seized from suspects and victims.

3. *Intelligence analysts.* Interpret the case evidence, digital or otherwise.

4. *Attorneys knowledgeable in this area.* Can readily interpret the rapidly developing area of computer and Internet law.

5. *Interviewers.* Extensively trained to ask the right questions of suspects, victims, and witnesses in order to find information and evidence needed to begin an investigation.

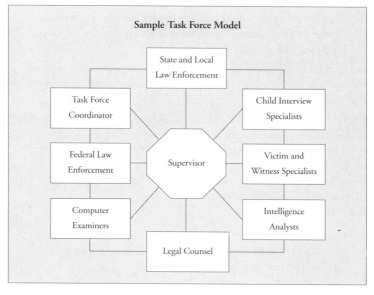

Figure 11-1. Various roles in a sample task force.

6. *Victim and witness specialists.* Help protect the welfare of child victims and maintain the integrity of the case.

— Many countries have established centers to serve as national collection points for Internet complaint information.

— In the United States, NCMEC serves this function.

LOCATING EVIDENCE

— The Internet Corporation for Assigned Names and Numbers performs many Internet managerial functions.

1. Most widely used services on the Internet follow a commonly accepted protocol specific to each service.

2. New protocols are usually first described in Request for Comments documents, formal papers that guide acceptance and adoption.

3. The major services used publicly on the Internet are listed in **Table 11-3**. Each area facilitates different types of communication, but all can foster CSE.

— To maintain compatibility among computer operating systems on the Internet, all existing and emerging services generally comply with the Transmission Control Protocol and/or Internet Protocol (IP).

— An Internet user must connect to a point-of-presence and obtain an IP address (a unique number that identifies a particular computer to others on the Internet).

— Users primarily connect via:

1. A modem or cable modem and an Internet service provider (ISP)

2. An online service provider

Table 11-3. Services Used Publicly on the Internet
— World Wide Web
— Internet relay chat (IRC)
— Electronic mail (e-mail)
— Usenet newsgroups
— File Transfer Protocol (FTP)
— Web-based chat (WBC)
— Messengers
— Peer-to-peer (P2P) networks

3. An Internet gateway provided by a corporate, government, library, education, or other computer network

— Users can typically be traced to their origin and identified. The primary concern is whether Internet records are available to provide the user's true identity. The likelihood of success increases with more complete and accurate information.

— Investigators must remember that the computer is an instrument used in the crime that has its own forensic value but is not the most important part of the investigation.

— When suspect identification is unclear or needs further supporting evidence, investigators rely on traditional investigative techniques (**Table 11-4**).

WORLD WIDE WEB

STRUCTURE

— The Web largely comprises billions of pages of information that provide everything: basic text, images, movies, music, and even software.

— Multiple pages form a Web site.

Table 11-4. "Traditional" Investigative Techniques
— Pretext calls
— Phone records
— Interview/interrogation
— Surveillance
— Trap and trace

1. Every page and element in the site has an Internet address, or Uniform Resource Locator (URL), that defines its location on the Web.

2. By following a hyperlink, users are taken to other locations to view other Web content.

3. A single Web page often comprises content from multiple states or countries, thereby complicating investigations.

HYPERTEXT TRANSFER PROTOCOL

— Hypertext Transfer Protocol is the essential means by which Web pages are transmitted for viewing.

— Information includes the Hypertext Markup Language programming code and the contents of other files related to the Web site being viewed.

— The code and files related to the Web site help investigators obtain information needed to identify the responsible party.

Problems Investigators Confront
— Information on who is responsible for Web content was formerly obtainable from log files and billing records, but the availability of free Web hosting and the complexity of Web pages complicate the process.

— Web page redirection may cause an Internet user to be unaware that the Web page address selected for viewing is not the one being viewed.

— Multiple suspects can be responsible for a single page or site, especially with a virtual community (often referred to as a Web club, e-group, or Web community).

Information Helpful to Investigators
— The minimum information needed to begin a Web site investigation is the URL of the site, the domain name, and the content's actual location.

— Ideally, obtain a copy of the Web site contents saved to a disk.

— An Internet investigation specialist can locate the registrant of the domain name, the host of the content, the ISP providing the Internet connection to the content (often the same as the host), and the ISP providing the domain name system entry for the Web site (**Figure 11-2**).

— Bogus registration information and frequently changing international hosts and connections pose challenges.

— An accurate URL must be obtained in a timely fashion.

— The Internet is a global entity, and a domain registrant can choose to register in a country other than the country code top-level domain (ccTLD) of the Web site's domain, so ccTLDs may not be entirely useful in locating an offender. A basic knowledge of ccTLDs is often helpful for investigators.

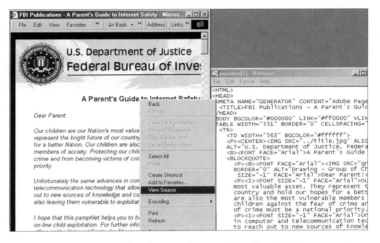

Figure 11-2. *Screen capture from the FBI Web site and the related HTML source code.*

INTERNET RELAY CHAT

— IRC is accessible to all Internet users.

— With appropriate software, users can connect to an IRC network server and then become connected to a particular network on which real-time chats with other users worldwide can be conducted in a chat room.

— Thousands of Internet chat rooms exist. Each is referred to within IRC as a channel.

— IRC also allows for private conversations and the private exchange of files through a file server (f-serve) without using e-mail.

— Major ISPs allocate server space to IRC and do not attempt to manage the content.

— For law enforcement officials to identify suspects on IRC, they must obtain:

1. The user's IRC nickname or online identity. However, IRC users can change their nicknames instantly.

2. The user's IP address and date, the time, and the time zone of the connection. However, complaining parties rarely have this information, so investigators may need to obtain more general infor-mation (eg, IRC network and server to which the suspect was connected or channel used by the suspect) to locate the suspect.

3. Anything saved to a disk is usually more useful than printed items.

Electronic Mail

— E-mail can be sent from and received within virtually any paid ISP account as well as via many free e-mail services.

— E-mail operates via its own set of protocols, with the most common being Simple Mail Transmission Protocol for sending and either Post Office Protocol or Internet Message Access Protocol for receiving e-mail.

— Most users view e-mail simply as an exchange of text and files between the addressed Internet users.

— E-mail information commonly seen by most users can be easily altered by using a spoof or remailer.

1. Most free e-mail accounts can be created using false user information or no information at all.

2. E-mail spam is a major plague of the Internet. Using spam e-mail as a delivery system for online security threats is considered a future threat to the Internet itself.

3. Tracking spam is difficult.

— Personally addressed e-mail can be traced by using the information related to e-mail transmission found in the message's header.

— With a copy of the message text but not the header information, the entire message can be obtained if that message remains stored on the mail server of the user's ISP.

— When in doubt, investigators should contact a properly trained investigator to help save the e-mail message to a disk, since a printout alone may be insufficient.

— Secure e-mail services are:

1. Designed to ensure the privacy of e-mail, thereby complicating the investigator's role.

2. Rarely used for child exploitation offenses.

USENET NEWSGROUPS

— Usenet newsgroups are virtual bulletin boards on which messages containing text and computer files are posted for public exchange.

— They are continuously updated by users worldwide and usually not monitored by host ISPs.

— Postings are maintained at ISPs for days or weeks and then may become available to download and trace to the user who posted the information, thereby providing valuable information to quick-acting investigators.

— People interested in the most heinous groups must pay for a private newsgroup service. Investigators fighting such newsgroups must also pay for this service.

— Posting and downloading content on newsgroups follows a protocol called Network News Transfer Protocol.

— Most newsgroup postings are easily traced by careful analysis of message header information.

1. ISPs may use different portions of a message header to determine the authoring account.

2. An investigator's best course of action is to provide the ISP with the entire message header if possible.

3. When the suspect posting is no longer available, knowledge of the poster's online identity, subjects' description of the postings, and the newsgroup to which the message is being posted can help locate the suspect.

FILE TRANSFER PROTOCOL

— Programs that use FTP are widely used by child pornographers.

— An FTP advertisement typically includes the IP address of the FTP server in addition to the username (ie, nickname) and password.

— Advertisers of FTP servers almost never charge for services and are usually individual users operating on their home, work, or school computer. Hundreds or thousands of servers probably operate secretly on the Internet.

— Once connected to an FTP server, users may upload and download files.

— Similar to an f-serve on IRC, FTP servers usually require users to upload images to receive credit to download others.

WEB-BASED CHAT (WBC)

— WBC, or chat, functions within a Web browser.

— WBC is easy to use compared with paid services provided by online service providers and free services like IRC.

— Chat within a Web browser is accomplished using small programs (known as applets or scripts) downloaded by the user to the computer browser.

— As in IRC, WBC identities or nicknames are easily changed.

— The evidence of chat rooms visited and messages sent and received is usually not logged.

— Unscrupulous users have flocked to IRC and WBC because a record of communication is not maintained unless intentionally kept by the sender or receiver.

— The computers of many suspects and victims might not show obvious signs of owners having used these services.

— WBC that incorporates Voice over IP (VoIP) allows users to talk to one another verbally rather than by typing.

— Tracing a user of WBC requires knowledge of the nickname or other online identity and a specific chat location, as one Web site can host thousands of chat rooms.

— Investigators must work quickly on WBC cases because the logs tracing offenders may expire within hours or days, if such logs are kept at all.

MESSENGERS

— Messengers are free, stand-alone software programs allowing users to instant message one another, create private or multiuser chat rooms, and send messages to and from properly equipped cellular telephones.

— Many functions of the messenger programs are being built into Internet-based game software that includes real-time chat between worldwide participants. Parents often do not recognize the potential harm of such games for their unsupervised children.

— The information needed to locate the user of a WBC or messenger program varies depending on the type of service used, but usually a nickname or other online identity is sufficient.

— One piece of information may be the difference between identifying or missing a targeted subject.

PEER-TO-PEER NETWORKS

— P2P networks are a relatively new variant of Internet programs.

— The term refers to 2 or more computers directly connected to one another without the aid of a central server.

— Internet P2P programs make file sharing easy for the masses.

— Programs that run on the major P2P networks can propagate child pornography and frustrate investigators.

1.   They show an icon only in the system tray on a Windows-based computer's clock rather than on the taskbar at the bottom center of the screen.

2.   Users are not typically connected via a central network but directly to one another so all users can share files. This grants an unlimited ability to download and upload computer files.

3. Criminal file transfers are difficult to trace without a direct connection between an investigator downloading and the person uploading these file transfers.

4. File transfers can occur only when users are connected to the program, so the amount of time available to look into a P2P complaint may be small.

5. Distributed P2P programs allow a user to simultaneously download a desired file from multiple users, thereby distributing the download among 2 or more computers.

— Investigators are especially urged to leave active, online investigations of P2P networks to properly trained professionals.

— Emerging threats:

1. Use of VoIP for Web-to-telephone calls

2. Rapid adoption of wireless technology. Improperly installed wireless home and business networks ripe for unauthorized access and abuse

3. Integration of computers and other home media

ONLINE SERVICE PROVIDERS (OSPS)

— OSPs make self-contained services available exclusively to subscribers.

— OSPs usually offer subscribers the ability to create user profiles that may contain either true or false information.

— OSPs make available paid services that provide some sort of verified information for investigators to use in locating a suspect.

— Maintaining the information is the services' prerogative, and few countries have laws requiring that these services maintain records useful to law enforcement officials. Some countries even have laws preventing the retention of such information or requiring the destruction of such information.

— Consider the long-term liaison relationship with online service providers and maintain decorum when dealing with them because a

positive relationship may make the difference in developing an effective case.

INTERNET PROTOCOL ADDRESS TRACING

— An IP address or domain name is usually available via public
databases from organizations known as Regional Internet Registries
(RIRs).

— There are 3 major RIRs responsible for registration on the Internet:

1. The American Registry for Internet Numbers is responsible for
    managing IP address numbers for the Americas and sub-Saharan
    Africa.

2. The Registrar for Internet Protocols in Europe is responsible for
    managing IP address numbers for Europe, the Middle East, the
    northern part of Africa, and parts of Asia.

3. The Asian-Pacific Network Information Center is responsible for
    managing IP address numbers for the Asian-Pacific region.

— Each registry has its own Internet Web page for referencing databases. Use the interface available at http://www.samspade.org, designed
by security expert Steve Blighty.

1. The site was originally set up to trace senders of spam and
    malicious computer hackers.

2. The site also provides other tools to Internet investigators and
    hobbyists.

IMPORTANCE OF TIME

— The chronology of events often links a particular suspect to a
particular crime in Internet investigations.

— The system known as Network Time Protocol is used to synchronize computer clock times in a network of computers, so most of the
times provided from ISP logs are accurate.

— This may not be the case when dealing with a victim's or suspect's
computer, or even the investigator's own computer. Most times pro-

vided by the computer to files are based on the system clock of that computer. Time of this clock may be set accidentally or intentionally by the user to display an incorrect time.

— It is critical for investigators to note the time displayed on the computer clock as well as any difference from the accurate, current time as part of a complete investigation.

— Time correction, as well as any correction based on time zone and possibly daylight savings time, can be used to compare critical events.

OTHER TECHNICAL CHALLENGES

— Starting or exiting Windows or any other operating system or even viewing or printing a computer file changes evidence integrity.

— Do not tamper with original evidence; rather, use working copies for analysis.

— A competent team leader and properly trained assistants should lead the search of a premise for computers and other related evidence. A certified computer examiner should be part of the search team.

— Searches conducted at a place of business or anywhere with potential innocent users should protect the work and privacy of the innocent.

— Information technology professionals at the suspect's place of employment can provide information and assistance once they are ruled out as potential suspects or accomplices.

— Seizure of the entire suspect computer system and related equipment is usually needed to maintain chain of custody.

— Look for low-tech items such as log books or notes containing online identities of the suspect or victims, account numbers leading to additional evidence, or even printed images or chat logs kept by the suspect for reference or remembrance.

— Even if the offender does not make these mistakes and enlists the use of high-tech protections (encryption or password protection), do not rely on the hope of cracking or guessing a password. Obtain the password from the suspect.

Undercover Technique

— Undercover (UC) operations are a primary investigative strategy for dealing with Internet crime when the technique is legally permitted.

— Many countries do not allow investigations of suspects who lack proper predisposition to commit a crime.

— An investigator who knowingly conducts unauthorized UC activity with subjects in countries in which such activity is illegal may be seen as infringing on national sovereignty.

— Carefully avoid issues of entrapment and remain cognizant of prevailing laws.

— If UC technique can be used, UC officers and agents may post as anyone on the Internet with relative ease and enjoy the same apparent anonymity as offenders.

— May include posing as a child and playing the role of a would-be victim, proactively identifying suspects, assuming the role of a fellow trader interested in child pornography, or pretending to be a molester with access to children who are available for sex.

— For UC investigations, use only computers that cannot be traced to government agencies or compromise other computers or networks.

— Be aware of potential harm from a computer virus, Trojan, or worm.

1. Must be proficient in using antivirus software and a network with a proper firewall or, preferably, a stand-alone computer with a personal firewall.

2. Update such programs continuously.

3. Scan all suspect files for viruses before opening.

— Use of a file name extension:

1. Most Windows-based computers do not show file extensions for known file types, but there are ways to configure computers to show all file extensions.

2. Many file extensions constitute a "danger list" (.exe, .vbs, .js, .asp, .shs, .scr, .com, .bat, .sys, .ovl, .prg, .mnu).

— Consider the file's source, the context in which the file was found, and any messages or other files associated with the suspect file.

OTHER INVESTIGATIVE TOOLS

— Typical law enforcement infrastructures were not designed for Internet pedophilia primarily because until relatively recently, child abuse was almost exclusively considered a local problem that required a local law enforcement response.

1. A key component of Internet pedophilia is local, yet the posted images are instantaneously global.

2. The same individuals who view their downloaded images while masturbating and fantasizing are likely to be a risk to children in the neighborhood, creating a local problem.

3. The proactive identification of such individuals is difficult and normally requires national or international police tactics.

— Most successful Internet victim identification investigations result from the collection and sharing of information from local sources (eg, seized computers, offender interviews). Many Internet child abuse images are part of large sets of images that can collectively furnish information about the location and time span of the abuse as well as other areas.

— EnCase is a computer forensics software program used in computer crime cases.

1. Fully integrated, Windows-based application

2. Performs all stages of the computer forensics investigation from the imaging of seized computer media, to the analysis and recovery of relevant information, to the verification and reporting of the recovered evidence

— See Chapter 14, Legal Approaches to Internet Cases, for a discussion of how to authenticate recovered data for accuracy and its use in prosecutions.

HOTLINES

— The Association of Internet Hotline Providers in Europe (IN-HOPE) coordinates Internet-related hotlines.

— INHOPE hotlines receive complaints from the public about alleged illegal Internet content, use of the Internet, or both.

— Procedures followed by INHOPE in handling these hotline calls:

1. When a hotline receives a report, the information is logged into the database.

2. Reports may be sent by e-mail, fax, letter, or telephone.

3. If the report is not submitted anonymously, confirmation of receipt is sent to the reporter.

4. Hotline staff members specially trained in assessing Internet content determine whether the material is illegal based on local laws.

5. If the material is legal, the report process is complete. It may be forwarded to a partner hotline for action.

6. If the material is illegal, hotline staff members begin an investigation to identify the origin.

7. If the illegal material is being hosted on a local server, the staff members involve local law enforcement officials, the relevant ISP, or both.

8. If the material is located on a server in a foreign country, INHOPE hotlines forward the report to the hotline in the country with the originating Web server.

9. If the country does not have an INHOPE hotline, INHOPE cooperates with various supranational organizations.

10. Criminal investigations are pursued by law enforcement officials.

11. The ISP is responsible for the timely removal of the content from their servers.

12. Once the hotline has notified law enforcement and the ISP the case is closed.

— INHOPE also operates working groups that address Internet content, the INHOPE Code of Practice, statistics, awareness and visibility, and membership issues.

— INHOPE uses the acronym REACT to describe the benefits of its network of hotlines: **R**eport-receiving mechanisms, **E**xpertise, **A**cceleration, **C**ontacts, and **T**rends. INHOPE reacts to reports that are received about alleged illegal content on the Internet, whereas law enforcement agencies are entitled to take a proactive approach, investigating content and pursuing perpetrators, so the roles of hotlines and law enforcement agencies are complementary.

REFERENCES

Federal Bureau of Investigation (FBI). A parent's guide to Internet safety. FBI Publications Web site. Available at: http://www.fbi.gov/publications/pguide/pguidee.htm. Accessed August 23, 2004.

Grubin D. *Sex Offending Against Children: Understanding the Risk*. London, England: Policing and Reducing Crime Unit; 1998. Police Research Series Paper 99.

Holland G. Victim identification project. Presented at: COPINE Presentation to European Parliament; December, 2003; Brussels, Belgium.

Whatis.com, Information Technology Computer Dictionary Web site. Available at: http://www.whatis.com. Accessed May 18, 2006

APPENDIX 26-1: GLOSSARY OF INTERNET-RELATED TERMS (WHATIS.COM, 2006)

American Registry of Internet Numbers (ARIN)—The organization responsible for the management of Internet Protocol (IP) address numbers for the Americas and sub-Saharan Africa.

Anti-virus software—A program that can detect known or potential viruses found on hard drives, on floppy disks, or in Internet traffic.

Asian-Pacific Network Information Center (APNIC)—The organization responsible for the management of IP address numbers for the Asia-Pacific region. There are 62 economies within the Asia-Pacific region, from Afghanistan in the Middle East to Pitcairn in the Pacific Ocean.

Bandwidth—The potential speed of data transmission on a communication medium.

Broadband—A communication medium that provides a wide band of frequencies to transmit information.

Browser—A program that allows the user to look at and interact with all the information found on the World Wide Web (WWW).

Cable modem—A device that enables the connection of a computer to a cable television line to receive, and possibly transmit, data at higher speeds.

Channel—A specific chat group found on Internet Relay Chat (IRC) similar to a chat room on a Web site or an online service provider.

Chat room—A Web site or part of a Web site found on an IRC channel or as part of an online service provider. A chat room provides a venue for communities of users with a common interest to communicate in real time.

Country code top-level domain (ccTLD)—The top-level domain name of an Internet address that identifies that domain generically as associated with a country. For example, in the domain name, "police.se," Sweden (ie, ".se") is the chosen cc TLD. Some ccTLDs can be inaccurate and misleading.

Cyberspace—The global community created by the interconnectedness of people through computers and the Internet.

Domain name—The labeling system that locates an organization or other entity on the Internet by a name that corresponds to an IP address. For example, the domain name "www.klpd.nl" locates an Internet address for "klpd.nl," which is the Netherlands National Police Agency at IP address 193.178.243.72.

Domain name system (DNS)—The manner in which Internet domain names are located and translated into IP addresses.

Download—The transmission of a file from one computer system to another, usually smaller computer system.

Digital Subscriber Line (DSL)—A broadband information system that brings high-bandwidth capacity to homes and businesses over ordinary telephone lines.

Electronic mail (e-mail)—The exchange of messages and sometimes file attachments via the Internet.

Encryption—The conversion of data into a form that cannot be easily understood by unauthorized people.

File name extension—An optional addition to a computer file name that describes the file's format in a suffix that usually consists of 3 characters (eg, .pdf, .doc, .jpg, .mpg, .avi).

File Transfer Protocol (FTP)—The IP for downloading and uploading files.

Firewall—Hardware or software located at a network gateway server that protects the resources of a private network from users of other networks.

Gateway—A network point that acts as an entrance to another network.

Generic top-level domain (gTLD)—The top-level domain name of an Internet address that identifies that address generically as associated with some domain class (eg, .com, .net, .org, .gov, .edu, .int, .mil). For example, in the domain name "www.fbi.gov," ".gov" is the chosen gTLD.

Header—In a newsgroup or e-mail message, the header is the portion of a transmission that is sent with the actual message and may identify the sender and other facts about the transmission.

Host—Any computer that has full, 2-way access (ie, transmit and receive) to other computers on the Internet.

Hosting—The business of housing, serving, and maintaining files for one or more Web sites. Also known as Web site hosting and Web hosting.

Hypertext Markup Language (HTML)—The set of symbols or codes inserted in a file that is intended for display on a Web browser.

Hypertext Transfer Protocol (HTTP)—The set of rules for exchanging files on the World Wide Web.

ICQ—A program used to notify users when friends and contacts are online on the Internet and allows the sending of messages, files, audio, and video to other users. Also known as I Seek You.

Instant message—The exchange of real-time messages with chosen friends or co-workers on the Internet.

Internet—A worldwide system of computer networks. A network of networks in which users at any one computer can, if they have permission, obtain information or other services from any other computer. Also known as the Net.

Internet Assigned Numbers Authority (IANA)—The organization under the Internet Architecture Board of the Internet Society that, under a contract from the US government, oversaw the allocation of IP addresses to Internet Service Providers. Partly because the Internet has become a global network, the US government has withdrawn its oversight of the Internet, which was previously contracted to IANA, and has lent support to an organization with global, nongovernment representation. The Internet Corporation for Assigned Names and Numbers (ICANN) has assumed responsibility for the tasks formerly performed by IANA.

Internet Corporation for Assigned Names and Numbers (ICANN)—The private, nongovernment, nonprofit corporation with responsibility for the services previously performed by the IANA.

Internet Message Access Protocol (IMAP)—A standard protocol for receiving e-mail.

Internet Protocol (IP)—The protocol by which data are sent from one computer to another on the Internet.

Internet Protocol (IP) address—A 32-bit number, which is usually expressed as 4 decimal numbers. Each decimal number represents 8 bits, which are used to identify senders and receivers of information across the Internet.

Internet Relay Chat (IRC)—A system for chatting within stand-alone software or within a Web browser.

Internet Service Provider (ISP)—A company that provides individual and corporate access to the Internet and other related services (eg, Web site building, hosting).

Link—A selectable connection on a Web page from a word, picture, or other information to another Web page or Internet object.

Modem—A device that modulates outgoing digital signals from a computer or other digital device into analog signals for a conventional, copper-twisted pair telephone line and demodulates the incoming analog signal and converts that signal to a digital signal for the digital device.

Network—A number of host computers interconnected by communication paths.

Network News Transport Protocol (NNTP)—The protocol for managing the messages posted on Usenet newsgroups.

Network Time Protocol (NTP)—Protocol used to synchronize computer clock times in a network of computers.

Newsgroup—A discussion about a particular subject that consists of messages posted and propagated through Usenet.

Online service provider—A service (eg, America Online) that has its own online, independent content rather than connecting users directly with the Internet. Most online service providers provide an Internet connection, in which case these providers function as ISPs as well.

Password—A sequence of characters used to determine whether a computer user requesting access to a computer system is an authorized user.

Peer-to-peer (P2P)—A communications model in which each party has the same capabilities and either party can send or receive information.

Personal firewall—A software application used to protect a single computer from intruders outside the network. Also known as a desktop firewall.

Point-of-presence (POP)—An access point to the Internet.

Post Office Protocol (POP3)—The most recent version of a standard protocol for receiving e-mail.

Protocol—A special set of communication rules.

Redirection—A technique for moving visitors to a Web page that differs from the address entered or followed by the user.

Regional Internet Registries (RIRs)—Entities that provide IP registration services. The 3 current RIRs are the American Registry for Internet Numbers (ARIN), the Registrar for Internet Protocols in Europe (RIPE), and the Asian-Pacific Network Information Center (APNIC).

Registrar for Internet Protocols in Europe (RIPE)—The organization responsible for the management of IP address numbers membership in Europe, the Middle East, northern Africa, and parts of Asia.

Remailer—An Internet site to which e-mail can be sent for forwarding to an intended destination but conceals the sender's e-mail address.

Request for Comments (RFC)—A formal document from the Internet Engineering Task Force (IETF) that resulted from committee drafting and subsequent review by interested parties.

Server—A computer program that provides services to other computer programs in the same network or different computers. The computer that the server program runs on is also referred to as a server.

Simple Mail Transport Protocol (SMTP)—A protocol primarily used in sending e-mail.

Social networking sites—Web sites where people become members to meet new people or stay connected with people they already know. Users can post pictures and profiles, but some users post false information to deceive others.

Spam—Unsolicited e-mail or other unwanted communications received on the Internet.

Spoof—To deceive for the purpose of gaining access to someone else's resources. For example, if a user fakes an Internet address to appear to be a different kind of Internet user, the user is spoofing.

System tray—A section of the taskbar in the Microsoft Windows desktop user interface that is used to display the clock and icons of certain programs. Some running programs appear only in the system tray.

Top-level domain (TLD)—Identifies the general part of the domain name in an Internet address. A TLD is either a generic TLD (gTLD) (eg, .com for commercial, .edu for educational) or a country code TLD (ccTLD) (eg, .nl for the Netherlands, .ie for Ireland).

Transmission Control Protocol (TCP)—A protocol used along with the IP to send data in the form of message units between computers over the Internet.

Trojan—A program in which a malicious or harmful code is contained. A Trojan appears to be harmless programming or data so that it can gain control and do damage (eg, ruining a hard disk). A Trojan may be redistributed as part of a virus.

Uniform Resource Locator (URL)—The address of a file (ie, resource) that is accessible on the Internet. For example, "http://www.fbi.gov/hq/cid/cac/innocent.htm" describes the Federal Bureau of Investigation's Innocent Images Web page. This URL indicates the page to be accessed with an HTTP (ie, Web browser) application located on a server named "www.fbi.gov." The specific file is in the directories of "/hq/cid/cac" and named "innocent.htm."

Upload—Transmission from one, usually smaller, computer to another computer.

Usenet—A collection of user-submitted messages about various subjects that are posted to servers on a worldwide network in which each subject collection of posted notes is known as a newsgroup.

Virtual community—A community of people sharing common interests, ideas, and feelings via the Internet or other collaborative networks.

Virus—A program or piece of a program usually disguised as something else, which causes an unexpected and usually undesirable event, usually seeking to contaminate only the host machine.

Voice over IP (VoIP)—A protocol for managing the delivery of voice information using the IP.

Web cam—A video camera, usually attached directly to a computer, whose image can be requested from a Web site. These can be live, continually providing new images or streaming video.

Web site—A collection of Web files regarding a particular subject that includes a beginning file called a home page. For example, the Web site for Ireland's National Police Service, An Garda Síochána, has the home page address of "http://gov.ie/garda."

Whois—A program that identifies registration information provided by the owner of any second-level domain name who has registered it with a Regional Internet Registry. Whois information can be bogus or incomplete.

World Wide Web (WWW)—All the resources and users found on the Internet using the HTTP.

Worm—A self-replicating virus that resides in active memory and duplicates itself with the intent of sending itself to other users.

Chapter 12

LEGAL ISSUES SPECIFIC TO PORNOGRAPHY CASES

Duncan T. Brown, Esq
Sharon W. Cooper, MD, FAAP

REGULATING CHILD PORNOGRAPHY

— Child pornography differs from adult obscenity; the normal test for adult obscenity outlined in *Miller v California* (1973) does not apply because compelling state interests make strict regulation permissible.

— Statutes defining child pornography must be narrowly tailored to fit state interests that allow its proscription (*R.A.V. v City of St. Paul,* 1992).

COMPELLING STATE INTERESTS
— Laws regulating child pornography are not content-neutral.

1. *First interest.* "Safeguarding the physical and psychological well-being of a minor" (*Globe Newspaper Co v Superior Court*, 1982). The right of the government to assume a greater duty to protect children from potential harm is a long-standing, legitimate role. The Supreme Court consistently recognizes this in cases of children exposed to obscenity and lewd material.

2. *Second interest.* Preventing future sexual abuse of children.

3. *Third interest.* The production and distribution of child pornography creates an economic motive for producing and distributing more pornography.

4. *Fourth interest.* Child pornography has no redeeming social value.

5. Additional concerns:

   A. Child molesters use child pornography as part of the grooming process (*United States v Acheson*, 1999).

   B. Child pornography serves to whet the appetite of child molesters and embolden them to commit acts of sexual assault on children.

NARROW DEFINITION

— The Supreme Court has interpreted the standard of narrow construction liberally to give states discretion in passing laws to address child pornography issues.

1. The First Amendment does not protect speech used by groups that promote or distribute child pornography. Any speech inciting a person to commit a criminal act in the near future is not protected by the First Amendment.

2. Whoever conspires to sexually exploit children receives the same treatment under the law as the coconspirator who commits the crime.

— Aspects of conspiracy: At least 2 people agree to commit an act, and one makes an overt act furthering that end (18 USCS § 371, 2001).

— Both the aider and abettor are criminally liable, regardless of whether an agreement was explicitly proved because the illegal act was actually completed with the defendant's aid (*Ianelli v United States*, 1975).

— Statutes criminalize the possession, production, and distribution of any pornographic material depicting a child in a sexually explicit manner (18 USC § 2252, 2001).

— Laws also prohibit images created by any means that combine elements of actual children with computer-generated images of prohibited child pornography, including images not solely composed of actual children.

— Understand the national and international aspects of the production and distribution of child pornography.

LEGAL ISSUES SPECIFIC TO COMPUTER EVIDENCE
See Chapter 14, Legal Approaches to Internet Cases.

MEDICAL EXPERT TESTIMONY
— The medical expert may have to explain to the jury why a child victim may disclose exploitation during the medical evaluation but consistently deny that pornographic images exist.

— Convey the message that victims are often so young that long-term impacts remain unknown.

1. The medical expert must be able to draw on literature regarding infant and toddler child sexual abuse to educate a jury about the potential harm done.

2. As school-aged children mature, anxiety about their images on the Internet has untold impact and contributes to frequent denials of the original events.

— The medical expert is often the final witness in a child sexual exploitation (CSE) case, providing an explanatory conclusion of all the facts presented.

— Understanding current research regarding why child pornographers collect images helps the medical expert explain generic offender dynamics.

— A sexual exploitation case may include a medical expert's testimony about a child the expert has never examined and whose diagnosis is drawn only from pictures placed in evidence.

— Careful testimony is needed to assist a jury in understanding the multiple forms of maltreatment present in some child pornography cases.

— The medical expert may also be needed to provide substantive evidence or serve to rehabilitate a child's damaged credibility after it has been attacked by a defense attorney (Myers & Stern, 2002).

1. Substantive testimony:

    A. Offer an opinion that the child has a diagnosis of child sexual abuse and/or CSE.

B. Use the phrase "consistent with [a specific diagnosis]" (eg, images are consistent with a child younger than 18 years).

C. Confine testimony to description of methods used to seduce or symptoms seen in sexually abused or exploited children as a group.

2. Rehabilitative testimony:

A. Address a child's delayed disclosure and abnormal behaviors indicative of other life circumstances, rather than abuse. Recantation is often misinterpreted as "finally telling the truth" but actually reflects family pressure on a child.

B. Scope is limited to specific points highlighted by the defense attorney.

C. Usually, it is restricted to a general review of the literature and the expert's experience with children as a group.

— Tips:

1. Avoid use of term "victim" because it sends the message to the jury that the expert believes the child was abused, which is for the jury to decide (Myers & Stern, 2002).

2. Avoid using the term "syndrome" because it infers that a specific diagnosis has been determined and causes the jury to feel no other option is available for their consideration (Myers & Stern, 2002).

TYPES OF EXPERT WITNESS TESTIMONY
— Background witness:

1. Educates judge or jury about general scientific information regarding relevant data on an abuse case.

2. Can explain the development of forensic pediatrics and the need to have knowledge in multiple areas to evaluate abuse.

— Case witness:

1. Reviews information specific to the case, including clinical medical records, videotaped interviews, mental health records, investigative reports, and the child protective services evaluation.

2.   Interprets data based on his or her knowledge of the literature and personal experience.

3.   Can draw conclusions that are case-specific and allow for testimony to reinforce information provided by the victim (Stern, 1997).

4.   May provide a more convincing argument for the victim status of the juvenile.

— Evaluating witness:

1.   Has knowledge of the background science and literature; has reviewed medical records, videotaped interviews, investigative reports, and other information; and has personally evaluated the child or juvenile.

2.   Can draw conclusions based on access to the greatest breadth of information.

3.   Has significant credibility; opinions are offered with the highest degree of confidence.

ELEMENTS OF TESTIMONY
— Medical history

1.   Specifically includes:

   A. *Method of disclosure.* Accidental disclosure? Excited utterance? In response to discovery of sexual props, etc? Delayed disclosure?

   B. *Content of disclosure.*

   C. *Consistency of the child's information.*

   D. *Sensory memory of the child.*

2.   See **Table 12-1** for core elements.

3.   See **Table 12-2** for pertinent questions to ask.

— Behavior

1.   Observed behavior overlaps with medical history (**Figure 12-1**).

Table 12-1. Core Elements in a Child Sexual Abuse History

— Who abused the child?

— What specifically happened?

— When did it occur?

— Where did the event(s) occur?

— How long did it continue in the child's life?

— What did the abuser say would happen if the child ever told?

Table 12-2. Questions Pertinent to Child Pornography

1. Were pornographic images shown to the child?

2. In what format were these images (photos, videos, computer images)?

3. Were these images of adults only or did they include children?

4. Did the suspect take any pictures of the child?

    A. If yes, in what format?

    B. What did the suspect say would happen to the photographs?

    C. Was the child alone or were there other children in the pictures?

5. Was the child offered or coerced into using drugs or alcohol before being sexually exploited?

6. Was the child instructed to do certain things to himself or herself, to another child, or to the suspect while the images were taken?

7. Was the child physically abused to coerce participation in the pornographic pictures or to ensure secrecy?

8. Was the child offered incentives for the exploitation?

9. Did the child witness incentives being given to a family member or caregiver in exchange for the child's participation?

10. Has the child ever seen the images? If so, where?

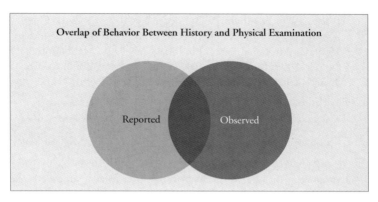

Figure 12-1. *There is overlap between the reported (medical history) and observed behavior (physical examination).*

2. Note abnormal behavior or changes in behavior such as emotional problems, depressive symptoms, low self-esteem, interpersonal problems, suicidal behavior, posttraumatic behaviors (see **Table 12-3**), substance abuse problems, increased sexualized behaviors, declining school performance, cognitive distortion, self-blame, and lack of interpersonal trust (Boney-McCoy & Finkelhor, 1995;

Table 12-3. Posttraumatic Stress Disorder (PTSD)

— Life-changing experience causing intense fear, helplessness, or horror (disorganized or agitated behavior)

— Reexperiencing the trauma events by intrusive thoughts, dreams, or trauma-specific reenactment

— Persistent avoidance of stimuli associated with the trauma

— Symptoms of increased arousal not present before the trauma (eg, insomnia, anger outbursts, inattentiveness, hypervigilance)

— Impairment of social, occupational, or other important areas of functioning

— Duration of symptoms for longer than 1 month

Briere, 1996; Friedrich, 1993; Friedrich et al, 1992, 2001; Gomes-Schwartz et al, 1990; Hibbard et al, 1990; Kilpatrick & Saunders, 1999; Lanktree et al, 1991; Lindblad et al, 1995; Mannarino & Cohen, 1996; McLeer et al, 1998; Ruggiero et al, 2000; Rust & Troupe, 1991; Stern et al, 1995; Wolfe & Birt, 1995).

— Physical examination

1. Is the least reliable of the testimonial elements.

2. See also Chapters 2, Victims and Offenders, and 7, Medical Issues.

SUMMARY OPINION

— Explain the number of child pornography images analyzed, the number of images consistent with children younger than the legal age of consent or that meet the legal definition of child pornography, and whether there existed images worthy of special mention because of the significant impact on the victim.

— When the actual child is present, detail the medical expert's role in making a medical diagnosis and prescribing treatment for the child.

— When the actual child is not present, offer corroborating information to confirm there is an actual child, determine the number of victims involved, or evaluate the abuse depicted.

REFERENCES

Boney-McCoy S, Finkelhor D. Psychosocial sequelae of violent victimization in a national youth sample. *J Consult Clin Psychol.* 1995;63:726-736.

Briere JN. A self-trauma model for treating adult survivors of severe child abuse. In: Briere JN, Berliner L, Bulkley J, Jenny C, Reid T, eds. *APSAC Handbook on Child Maltreatment.* Thousand Oaks, Calif: Safe Publications; 1996:140-157.

18 USCS § 2252 (2001).

18 USCS § 371 (2001).

Friedrich WN. Sexual victimization and sexual behavior in children: a review of recent literature. *Child Abuse Negl.* 1993;17:59-66.

Friedrich WN, Grambsch P, Damon L, et al. The child sexual behavior inventory: normative and clinical findings. *Psychol Assess.* 1992;4:303-311.

Friedrich WN, Dittner CA, Action R, et al. Child sexual behavior inventory: normative, psychiatric and sexual abuse comparisons. *Child Maltreat.* 2001;6:37-49.

Globe Newspaper Co v Superior Court, 457 US 596 (1982).

Gomes-Schwartz B, Horowitz JM, Cardarelli AP. *Child Sexual Abuse: The Initial Effects.* Thousand Oaks, Calif: Sage Publications; 1990.

Hibbard RA, Ingersoll GM, Orr DP. Behavior risk, emotional risk, and child abuse among adolescents in a nonclinical setting. *Pediatrics.* 1990;86:896-901.

Ianelli v United States, 420 US 770 (1975).

Kilpatrick DG, Saunders BE. *Prevalence and Consequences of Child Victimization: Results From the National Survey of Adolescents.* Charleston: National Crime Victims Research & Treatment Center, Department of Psychiatry & Behavioral Sciences, Medical University of South Carolina; 1999. No 93-IJ-CX-0023.

Lanktree CB, Briere J, Zaidi L. Incidence and impact of sexual abuse in a child outpatient sample: the role of direct inquiry. *Child Abuse Negl.* 1991;15:447-453.

Lindblad F, Gustafsson PA, Larsson I, Lundin B. Preschoolers' sexual behavior at daycare centers: an epidemiological study. *Child Abuse Negl.* 1995;19:569-577.

Mannarino AP, Cohen JA. Abuse-related attributions and perceptions, general attributions, and locus of control in sexually abused girls. *J Interpers Violence.* 1996;11:162-180.

McLeer SV, Dixon JF, Henry D, et al. Psychopathology in non-clinically referred sexually abused children. *J Am Acad Child Adolesc Psychiatry.* 1998;47:1326-1333.

Miller v California, 413 US 15 (1973).

Myers JEB, Stern P. Expert testimony. In: Myers JEB, Berliner L, Briere J, Hendrix CT, Jenny C, Reid TA, eds. *The APSAC Handbook on Child Maltreatment*. 2nd ed. Thousand Oaks, Calif: Sage Publications; 2002:386-395.

R.A.V. v City of St. Paul, 505 US 377,383-384 (1992).

Ruggiero KJ, McLeer SV, Dixon JF. Sexual abuse characteristics associated with survivor psychopathology. *Child Abuse Negl*. 2000; 24:951-964.

Rust JO, Troupe PA. Relationships of treatment of child sexual abuse with school achievement and self-concept. *J Early Adolesc*. 1991; 11:420-429.

Stern AE, Lynch DL, Oates RK, O'Toole BI, Cooney G. Self esteem, depression, behaviour and family functioning in sexually abused children. *J Child Psychol Psychiatr*. 1995;36:1077-1089.

Stern P. *Preparing and Presenting Expert Testimony in Child Abuse Litigation: A Guide for Expert Witnesses and Attorneys*. Thousand Oaks, Calif: Sage Publications; 1997.

United States v Acheson, 195 F3d 645,649 (11th Cir 1999).

Wolfe VV, Birt J. The psychological sequelae of child sexual abuse. *Adv Clin Child Psychol*. 1995;17:233-263.

Chapter 13

LEGAL CONSIDERATIONS IN PROSTITUTION CASES

The Honorable Ernestine S. Gray
Susan S. Kreston, JD, LLM
Bernadette McMenamin, AO

LAWS AND PENALTIES

— Victimized children's attachment to their pimps and the nonco-operation that results create difficulties in investigations and prosecutions.

— The federal government and most states have laws against prostituting children.

— Laws usually target the conduct of the economic exploiter and/or pimp but ignore the culpability of the sexual molester and/or john.

— Penalties differ significantly for crimes labeled "prostitution" versus those called "child sexual abuse."

1. *Patrons* are often specifically excluded from legislation on the prostitution of children.

2. When patrons are included, the penalty is generally lighter than for a molester prosecuted under traditional child sexual abuse laws.

3. Cases are shuffled among juvenile, vice, family, and criminal divisions of police departments because sexual molesters are usually extrafamilial and the victims tend to be teenagers; therefore, consent issues are involved (Walsh & Fassett, 1994).

4. Many cases and children are lost.

5. Even when adjusting for all other variables, crimes against teenagers carry lighter sentences than crimes against other victims (Finkelhor & Ormrod, 2001).

— State laws pertaining to prostituted children:

1. Most state laws do not specifically focus on patrons but address criminal liability. Crimes are usually handled as a summary or misdemeanor offense (Klain, 1999).

2. Laws dealing with individuals who operate or manage the prostitution of children address crime in terms of pimping, pandering, procuring, profiting, or promoting prostitution and reflect various degrees of protection based on the child's age (younger children receive more protection) (Klain, 1999).

3. Additional state laws impose penalties on individuals who aid or abet the prostitution of children (Klain, 1999).

— Federal laws applying to the prostitution of children can be found in the Mann Act (18 USC section 2421, et seq. Section 2423):

1. These laws specifically address the prostitution of children as well as transportation and travel with intent to engage in criminal sexual activity.

2. Section 2423(a) targets criminal culpability of the pimp and allows for prosecution of offenders who knowingly transport a minor across state lines with the intent to prostitute.

3. Section 2423(b) allows for prosecution of patrons who cross state lines with the intent of prostituting a child, regardless of whether exploitation actually occurs.

TRIAL CONSIDERATIONS
CHARGING AND PRETRIAL DECISIONS
— Must determine:

1. If sufficient, admissible evidence exists to prove the defendant's guilt beyond a reasonable doubt.

2. Who will be charged with the crime and what safeguards are needed to ensure defendants do not leave the jurisdiction.

3.   When prosecution is possible, whether prosecution should take
       place in a federal or state venue, or both.

— Because victims may be unwilling to testify (due to feelings of
loyalty to or fear of pimp, fear their sexual history will be revealed,
etc), prosecutor should request a rape shield hearing to obtain a ruling
from the court to restrict the evidence to include only the sexual
history relevant to the case (Federal Rule of Evidence 412; Myers,
1997, suppl 2002).

— A victim witness advocate may serve as a bridge and buffer between
victim and prosecutor if victim has hostile feelings toward law enforcement officers and prosecutors.

— Consider other attendant crimes, including child abuse or sex
crimes, violence charges, production and distribution of pornography,
aggravated sexual abuse, sexual abuse of a minor or ward, racketeering,
money laundering, tax fraud, and accessory and/or accomplice liability.

— Relevant factors to be considered before trial:

1.   Convenience for the victim and witnesses

2.   Docket load

3.   Speed of trial

4.   Jurisdiction with best resources for prosecution

JURY SELECTION

— An ideal juror empathizes with children, feels comfortable with
hearing and believing the testimony of children, holds adults accountable for their actions, is aware of this type of child abuse, and is
committed to the rule of law.

— A theme should be developed and carried throughout the trial.

— Points to cover when educating the jury during voir dire (see also
Chapter 14, Legal Approaches to Internet Cases):

1.   Witness credibility

2.   Appearance, conduct, and/or character of witness

3. Expert testimony

4. Potential juror biases or prejudices

— Case-specific facts:

1. Victim identification and history

2. Victim recantation of disclosure

3. Juror's attitude toward adult prostitution

OPENING STATEMENT

— This statement is the first opportunity to present the prosecution's theory of the case and provide the jury with the theme to be used throughout the trial and during the closing argument.

— Begin to personalize the victim. Refer to the child by name and show the child as a unique human being who has been violated.

— Tips:

1. Keep opening statement brief and provide only the blueprint of the evidence to be presented.

2. If there are problems with the case, mention them up front.

3. Do not oversell the case or promise more than will be delivered.

4. Ask the jury to return the only just and true verdict possible after the evidence is presented: Guilty as charged.

CASE IN CHIEF

— Recognize the case as a child abuse situation.

— Create strategies to deal with a less-than-sympathetic victim whose credibility may be an issue for the jury.

— Confirm the existence and reality of prostituted children's experiences.

— Victim testimony:

1. Determine whether the victim is cooperative. If not, explain the reasons for the uncooperative attitude to the jury.

2. If the victim denies previously acknowledged events, impeach the denials with prior inconsistent statements.

3. If the child refuses to testify, hearsay exceptions may allow for admission of prior statements (eg, excited utterance, prior identification, present sense impression, or medical diagnosis and treatment) (see Chapter 14, Legal Approaches to Internet Cases).

4. Explore how the child became involved with prostitution so the jury has a full picture of what the victim experienced.

— Law enforcement testimony:

1. Provides background information regarding the prostitution of children.

2. Explains the details of the specific case.

3. Assures jurors that the law enforcement officers involved took the case seriously while investigating.

4. Allows for impression management. Investigators inform jurors of the time and effort put forth by law enforcement officers investigating the case, which conveys their commitment.

— Other expert witness testimony:

1. *Child sexual abuse accommodation syndrome expert.* Called to educate jury about the counterintuitive aspects of the sexually exploited child's behavior. Includes issues such as entrapment, accommodation, recantation, and the child's feelings of helplessness to help jurors understand the psychology of a child victim and why the child could not simply leave the situation.

2. *Offender typologist.* Testifies as to how exploiters select victims and look for children who will not tell or who are unlikely to be believed if they do. Includes information on how exploiters initially engage children, groom them for abuse, and ensure secrets will be kept or not believed when they are disclosed (see also Chapter 2, Victims and Offenders).

3. These witnesses are most effective before the child testifies; the prosecutor can then show how the child's and offender's behaviors are consistent with the expert testimony.

Closing Argument

—Opening close:

1. Reference the theme and theory of the case.

2. Summarize the evidence and how it proves each element of the case beyond a reasonable doubt.

3. Present the strongest points first but also address weaknesses.

4. Dispose of defenses by addressing claims of innocence in light of the evidence and common sense.

— Rebuttal argument:

1. Note the defense's arguments and prepare to address them.

2. Respond to points in order of importance.

3. Correct any misstatements of fact and address questions raised regarding how things were or were not done in the investigation.

4. Expose the defense strategy.

5. Reinforce and recapitulate the strongest points, finishing with a definitive concluding statement.

6. Refer to jury instructions.

Sentencing

— Judge's pronouncement should reflect the community's negative attitude toward child abuse as well as the seriousness of and harm caused by the defendant's conduct.

— Punishment should be consistent with that received for other types of child sexual abuse.

— Prosecutor should be prepared to refute dubious claims in mitigation.

— Prosecutor should also create and protect a record that supports sentencing.

— Aspects:

1. Defendant may be designated as a sexual offender for the purposes of community registration and notification under the local equivalent of Megan's Law.

2. Defendant may have to make restitution to the victim to defray the costs of counseling or rehabilitation expenses.

3. Defendant may forfeit property used in the criminal activity.

JUVENILE COURT ISSUES

— The main participants and their roles in the modern juvenile court process are detailed in **Table 13-1.**

— The juvenile court system is ill equipped to deal with the prostitution of children.

1. Deficiencies result from the adult system's failure to use the legal tools already existing, such as the enforcement of laws in situations that involve the prostitution of children, because these laws were designed to protect minors from sexual mistreatment.

2. Aggressive enforcement would discourage adults from exploiting children.

Table 13-1. Participants and Their Roles in the Modern Juvenile Court

— *The judge.* Generally has more power, by tradition and law, than judges in other arenas, granting the judge freedom to craft decisions that are creative and appropriate

— *The child's attorney.* Charged with advancing the best legal interest of the child, whether the case involves a delinquency (ie, criminal) charge or an abuse and/or neglect situation

— *A guardian ad litem, a court-appointed special advocate (CASA), or another person charged with a similar role.* Looks after the child's general interest (ie, social, psychological, and so on) more broadly than the child's attorney

— *The parents' attorney.* Looks after the parents' interest in an abuse and/or neglect case

— *The prosecutor.* Performs the role of prosecuting the accused juvenile (ie, in a delinquency case) or of petitioning for the child's removal from the home or for the termination of the parents' parental rights (ie, in an abuse and/or neglect case)

---

3. The judicial response to children who have engaged in prostitution is often insufficient or inappropriate.

— Perceptions to be overcome:

1. Victims can get out of the situation if they so choose.

2. Girls are difficult for service providers to work with.

3. Judges believe they have no option other than incarceration for runaway children involved in prostitution.

4. A child involved in the "adult" behavior of prostitution is no longer a child worthy of the protection accorded other children.

5. Laws designed to protect children from sexual abuse are not applicable to prostituted children cases.

6. Prostituted people are bad, outcasts, or those who make poor choices rather than victims.

7. Teenagers in particular are bad or different.

— Changes needed:

1. Enforcement of existing criminal law against the customers of and other adults who benefit from the prostitution of children.

2. Creation of model statutes to address insufficiencies of laws related to the definition of crime and punishment so that johns and pimps face significantly more severe consequences.

3. Expanded treatment services that are culturally competent and developmentally appropriate.

4. Increased number of shelters for runaway and homeless youths and provision of more options for placement.

5. Community awareness of and intolerance for sexual abuse of children in situations involving prostitution that is equivalent to society's response to child sexual abuse in other situations.

6. Mentors to provide healthy role models to enable children to perceive alternatives for their lives.

7.   Opportunities for these children to participate in athletic and other constructive events.

8.   Appropriate work opportunities for children.

INTERNATIONAL RESOURCES FOR CHILD SEX TOURISM CASES

— Globalization is considered the major force behind the rapid international increase and expansion of the child sex trade.

— Many Western countries have begun to crack down on child sex offenders.

1.   Enact stronger laws

2.   Increase law enforcement efforts

3.   Tighten employment screening measures

4.   Conduct police checks

5.   Compile and maintain sex offender databases to track offenders

— End Child Prostitution in Asian Tourism Campaign: Its aim is to raise international awareness of the problem, build active grassroots advocacy groups, effect a global network, and encourage governmental organizations and communities to implement laws and policies to stop child sexual exploitation.

— Tourism incentives:

1.   *Child Wise Tourism.* A training and network development program seeking to build partnerships among government agencies, nongovernmental agencies, and the tourism industry to protect children from sexual exploitation.

2.   *Association of Southeast Asian Nations Regional Think Tank.* Organizes venues for communication among government, national tourism authorities, travel industry representatives, and child protection agency officials to develop and strengthen working relationships and stress the reality of the need to prevent child sex tourism.

3. *Code of Conduct.* Designed to raise awareness of child sex tourism among European tour operators, their local partners in tourist destinations, and travelers.

4. *Youth Career Initiative.* Includes a basic course in the hospitality industry aimed at empowering young people considered at risk specifically for sexual abuse to make choices about their future, provides opportunities to enter the workforce in the tourism industry, and teaches young people life skills.

REFERENCES

18 USC § 2241.

18 USC § 2243.

18 USCA § 2423 (a).

18 USCA § 2423 (b).

Federal Rule of Evidence 412.

Finkelhor D, Ormrod R. *Offenders Incarcerated for Crimes Against Juveniles.* Washington, DC: US Dept of Justice, Office of Justice Programs, Office of Juvenile Justice and Delinquency Prevention; 2001.

Klain EJ. *Prostitution of Children and Child-Sex Tourism: An Analysis of Domestic and International Responses.* Alexandria, Va: National Center for Missing & Exploited Children; 1999:2.

Myers JEB. *Evidence in Child Abuse and Neglect Cases.* 3rd ed. New York, NY: Aspen Law and Business; 1997(suppl 2002):101-121, 557.

Walsh W, Fassett B. Juvenile prostitution: an overlooked form of child sexual abuse. *The APSAC Advisor;* 1994;7(1):9.

Legal Approaches to Internet Cases

Susan S. Kreston, JD, LLM
John Patzakis, Esq

Search and Seizure Issues

— Traditional tools used in criminal investigations, such as the search warrant, must be adapted to respond to crimes involving the Internet. Prosecutors are specifically encouraged to review the recently enacted Patriot Act of 2001.

Search Warrants

— Warrants must contain a detailed, specific description of the place to be searched and the person(s) or thing(s) to be seized and must be supported by probable cause.

— Items to be seized must be defined with sufficient detail so as to limit the executing officer's discretion in deciding what will be seized.

Background Information

— Introductory paragraph gives the affiant's training and experience in investigating child sexual exploitation (CSE).

— List the affiant's present rank and assignment, areas of responsibility, length of experience as a law enforcement officer, training and work experience in CSE, training and work experience in the area of computers, including consultation with other law enforcement officers trained in computer investigations, and any other relevant information.

— The affiant may rely on the expertise of others.

— Include information explaining the Internet and computer technologies in search warrant application. Do not assume the judge is up to date with the latest technologies or jargon.

Probable Cause

— Probable cause is established through an affidavit in support of the warrant, setting out the factual basis for the warrant application.

— The judge must decide whether there is a fair probability that contraband or evidence of a crime will be found (*United States v Garcia*, 1993; *United States v Pitts*, 1993; *United States v Ricciardelli*, 1993; *United States v Simpson*, 1998).

— Affidavits supporting the warrant application should be specifically incorporated by reference into the warrant.

— Establish the following:

1. There is a computer physically located in a particular location.

2. The computer contains evidence of, or was used to commit, a crime.

— Explain the means to track the suspect's usage of the Web site for determining whether there are downloaded child pornography images.

— Do not rely solely on the Web site's personal and billing information to establish identity. Ensure the account(s) was not set up by someone impersonating the suspect.

— Establish a nexus between the child pornography and the computer to be searched.

Drafting the Warrant

— Undercover communications with the suspect via the Internet often furnish probable cause for believing the suspect's computer contains child pornography and other evidence of distribution and receipt.

— Warrant can list the title of each image and describe its contents so the reviewing magistrate can determine legality.

— Printed copies of the images can be placed in sealed envelopes for the magistrate to review.

— Include accompanying e-mail messages and titles of images if they provide evidence concerning the suspect's knowledge that they feature children engaged in sexually explicit conduct. Internet relay chat channels and newsgroups are typically named to correspond to the users' interest (see Chapter 11, Investigating Cyber-Enticement).

— Note any evidence demonstrating the suspect is a candidate likely to fit the behavioral characteristics identified.

— Child pornography warrants typically authorize the seizure of all images of child pornography, but they should specifically define the meaning of the term. When the suspect is downloading child pornography files from, or uploading files to, a newsgroup, include descriptions and explanations.

— The Fourth Amendment does not generally require the specific search methodology be spelled out in the warrant application (*United States v Hill*, 2004).

Expert Opinion

— The key is to set forth the characteristics and mode of operation of pedophiles, specific facts as to how the defendant demonstrates those characteristics, and support for any conclusions that the suspect fits into that class of persons.

— An expertise component should explain, in a case-specific manner, why or how particular characteristics apply to the suspect (*United States v Lamb*, 1996).

— This component supplements the probable cause developed in the affidavit or addresses potential staleness issues (*United States v Anderson*, 1999).

Additional Considerations in Describing Items to Be Seized

— Remember "traditional" types of child molestation evidence when drafting a search warrant.

— Seek physical and forensic evidence from the victim, suspect, and crime scene.

1. Special equipment, such as luminol lights, may be needed to search for some of the items properly and thoroughly.

2. When executing a warrant, look for evidence corroborating the child's account of the abuse (**Table 14-1**).

3. Items subject to seizure depend on the nature of the investigation.

PARTICULARITY

— An entire class of items may be seized if the warrant is sufficiently particular, establishing probable cause that will support seizure of the entire class, and a more precise description is not possible.

— When detailed particularity is impossible, generic language, if it particularizes the types of items to be seized, is permitted (*United States v Horn*, 1999; *United States v Layne*, 1995).

Table 14-1. Physical and Forensic Evidence to Consider in Child Molestation Cases

PHYSICAL EVIDENCE

— Sexual devices
— Lubricants
— The child's clothing/underwear
— Bondage and discipline paraphernalia
— Adult pornography
— Any items that could be used to abuse or exploit the child sexually or physically

FORENSIC EVIDENCE

— Blood
— Blood spatter
— Semen
— Vaginal fluid
— Urine
— Hair
— Fiber evidence
— Chemical evidence

— Typographical statutory citation errors may be rendered harmless if the full content of the statute is put into the warrant.

— Overbreadth issues arise when the warrant is too broad and includes items that should not be seized.

ANTICIPATORY WARRANTS

— Become effective on the happening of a future event

1. Anticipatory warrants should be upheld when supported by probable cause and conditions precedent are clearly set forth in the warrant or its supporting affidavit.

2. They differ from traditional warrants in that they are unsupported by probable cause for believing that the items to be seized are at the place to be searched at the time the warrant is issued (*United States v Loy*, 1999; *United States v Rowland*, 1998).

3. They must be supported by probable cause at the time of issuance.

4. They must establish probable cause to believe the contraband will be there when the warrant is executed.

5. The triggering event is typically future delivery, sale, or purchase of contraband.

6. If the triggering event does not occur, the warrant is void.

7. A warrant that does not identify the triggering event is fatally defective.

8. If the place to be searched is not the site of the delivery, sale, or purchase of the contraband, added facts must be offered to support probable cause to believe contraband will be taken to the location to be searched.

GOOD FAITH

— Even if no nexus is established, the good faith exception may allow for the admissibility of seized item(s) (*United States v Loy*, 1999; *United States v Rowland*, 1998).

— Requires that the officer acted in reasonable reliance on a warrant issued by a detached and neutral magistrate and was unaware of the lack of support by probable cause despite a magistrate's authorization.

STALENESS

— An expert should address whether a particular suspect is likely to keep contraband for long periods of time.

— The age of information supporting a warrant application is a factor in determining probable cause.

1. If the information is too old, it is stale and probable cause may no longer exist.

2. Age alone is not the sole determinant of staleness—consider the nature of the crime and type of evidence.

3. Lapse of time is less important when the suspected criminal activity is continuing in nature and when property is not likely to be destroyed or dissipated (*United States v Horn*, 1999).

— Those who deal in pornography treat materials as valuable commodities, sometimes regarding them as collections and retaining them in secure but available places for extended periods of time (Lanning, 2001). An appropriate reference to expert opinion that child pornography collectors retain their collections for long periods of time can overcome staleness of information.

EXCEPTIONS TO WARRANT REQUIREMENT

Plain View Exception

Applies to seizure of electronic evidence if officers are in a lawful position to observe evidence and its incriminating character is immediately apparent.

Consent Exception

— Consent from the party whose computer is being searched may eradicate the need for a search warrant, provided the consent is voluntary and not coerced.

— A warrantless search must be executed with the permission of an authorized party.

— Consent searches can raise multiple issues depending on the parties involved.

— When a third party gives consent, the question of whether that party had common authority over the object of the search and, as a result, the authority to consent to the search arises.

— A spouse can usually give consent to a search for evidence and seizure of a computer if the computer is used by both spouses. Exception is when 1 spouse has excluded the other from using the computer or from entering certain files within the computer by the use of encryption or passwords known only to him or her.

— Parents of minors generally can consent to a search by law enforcement of a computer used by the minor.

1. Exception: a minor maintained an expectation of privacy by virtue of being emancipated under state law for a particular purpose.

2. Parents of an adult child who lives with them generally cannot consent to a search by law enforcement of the adult child's computer unless the parent is a co-user of the computer.

— Apparent authority of the consenting individual and the police's reasonable belief in that apparent authority may suffice as valid consent.

— Consent to search given after an illegal entry is tainted and invalid under the Fourth Amendment (*United States v Hotal*, 1998).

— Employees' expectation of privacy in their workplace computers depends on the notification given to the employees by management on this issue.

Exigent Circumstances Exception

— Exception comprises urgency; the amount of time needed to obtain a warrant under particular facts of the investigation; likelihood evidence would be destroyed, concealed, or altered; danger to officers or others, whether the target knows law enforcement is coming to crime scene; the nature of evidence and its susceptibility to destruction by remote "kill" switches or other means of destroying or concealing the evidence; and whether the target computer is part of a network of computers that would facilitate the transfer of contraband to other computers outside the jurisdiction of the warrant.

— When police fear the destruction of evidence, they can enter the home of an unknown suspect if (1) there is clear evidence of probable cause, (2) it is for a serious crime, (3) evidence destruction is likely, (4) it is limited to minimum intrusion needed to prevent destruction of evidence, and (5) it is supported by clearly defined indications of an exigency not subject to police manipulation or abuse (*United States v Anderson*, 1998).

— A no-knock warrant allows police to enter private premises without knocking and without identifying themselves.

Private Searches
— The Fourth Amendment does not apply to nongovernmental actors unless agency principals are present. Note that law enforcement may not use civilians to act on its behalf without making those persons subject to the same rules as law enforcement personnel.

— Investigators may obtain a warrant based on the private search if the scope of the private search is not expanded (*United States v Grimes*, 2001).

Probation and Parole Searches
— Government may closely supervise probationers and impinge on their privacy more than for the general public.

— An anonymous tip may form the basis for a warrantless search of a parolee's residence if it is suitably corroborated.

CHARGING AND PRETRIAL CONSIDERATIONS
DEFINING CHILD PORNOGRAPHY
— Federal law prohibits minors from engaging in sexually explicit conduct (see definition, Chapter 1, Overview).

— Evaluate pictures to determine the intent of the photographer.

PROVING SCIENTER
Must prove that the defendant knew the person in a visual depiction was a minor.

STATUTES OF LIMITATION ISSUES
Crimes against children committed after April 2003 have no statute of limitation, whereas those committed before that date are governed by the law in place when the act was committed.

JURISDICTION
— Usually, there is one jurisdiction in child abuse cases and multiple in child pornography, especially if images were distributed over the Internet.

— Consider differences between federal and state child pornography laws, federal and state case law, and penalties for the offense; experience of prosecutors and resources of their offices; admissibility of prior uncharged acts; and the existence of civil commitment statutes.

NUMBER OF COUNTS AND IMAGES TO CHARGE
— Do not charge more offenses than needed to reflect the nature and extent of the criminal conduct and provide a basis for an appropriate sentence.

— Charges are not filed to exert leverage in plea negotiations and not abandoned to reach a plea agreement.

— Offenses may be charged to strengthen the case or provide a tactical advantage.

— Can charge 1 count for each computer image file possessed by the defendant that contains a visual depiction of a minor engaged in sexually explicit conduct.

— Each count must be proved beyond a reasonable doubt.

— Decide how many images to charge. If only prepubescent child images are charged, this eliminates any potential mistake of fact defense and reinforces to the jury that prosecutorial discretion is being properly exercised.

ADDITIONAL AND/OR ALTERNATIVE CHARGES

Consider charges of molestation, and so on, when factually appropriate.

VICTIM ISSUES

— Be prepared to prove an image is of a real person and that the person is a minor.

— If the child is a known person, consider victim issues in making major case decisions.

— Consult with the Federal Bureau of Investigation's Innocent Images Task Force, which has trained child interview specialists available to assist with or conduct victim interviews.

DISCOVERY ISSUES

— The state should not surrender child pornography without a final court order directing this action.

— The defense's viewing of child pornography should be restricted to a location in a government office.

— Protect the defense's privacy to ensure privileged communications.

— No notice is given to the state concerning the identity of potential defense experts.

— Follow the most recent state laws.

AUTHENTICATION OF RECOVERED DATA FOR ACCURACY

COMPUTER EVIDENCE

— Computer data are defined legally as documents. Documents and writings must be authenticated before they may be introduced into evidence.

1. Such data can be easily altered without proper handling.

2. The proponent of evidence normally carries the burden of offering sufficient evidence to authenticate documents or writings, and electronic evidence is no exception.

— Admission of computer evidence, typically as active text or graphic image files, is accomplished without using specialized computer forensic software.

— Federal Rule of Evidence 901(a) provides that the authentication of a document is "satisfied by evidence sufficient to support a finding that the matter in question is what the proponent claims."

— No specific requirements or set procedures exist for the authentication of chat room conversation logs, but courts generally favor having the facts and circumstances of the creation and recovery of the evidence according to Rule 901(a).

THE RECOVERY PROCESS

— When direct testimony is unavailable, a document may be authenticated through circumstantial evidence.

— Examiners must provide competent and sufficient testimony to connect the recovered data to the crime.

— Examiners need not detail how each function of cloning software works to provide sufficient testimony regarding the process.

— A strong working familiarity of how the program is used and what the cloning process involves is necessary when seeking to introduce evidence recovered by the program.

— Examiners should conduct their own software testing and validation to confirm that the program functions as advertised.

CHALLENGES TO FOUNDATION MUST HAVE FOUNDATION

— Expert testimony to rebut contentions may be needed.

— Normally, courts disallow challenges to the authenticity of computer-based evidence absent a specific showing that the computer data in question may not be accurate or genuine.

— Unsupported claims of possible tampering or overlooked exculpatory data are common and met with considerable skepticism by the courts.

Validation of Computer Forensic Tools
— Question the reliability of the computer program that generated or processed the computer evidence.

— The proponent of the evidence must testify as to the validity of the program or programs used in the process.

Daubert/Frye Standard
— Basic elements of the *Daubert* analysis (*Daubert v Merrell Dow Pharmaceuticals*, 1993; *Frye v United States*, 1923):

1. Whether a "theory or technique ... can be (and has been) tested."

2. Whether it "has been subjected to peer review and publication."

3. Whether, in respect to a particular technique, there is a high "known or potential rate of error."

4. Whether the theory or technique enjoys "general acceptance" within the "relevant scientific community."

— Courts favor commercially available and standard software. Widespread adoption of the software by the computer forensics community is a crucial factor in authentication.

— Any testing should be meaningful and objective, as well as subject to the same peer review as the tools and processes being analyzed.

— No ideal amount of published testing exists.

Computer Forensics as an Automated Process
— Federal Rule of Evidence 901(b) provides a presumption of authenticity to evidence generated by or resulting from a largely automated process or system shown to produce an accurate result.

— In more complex computer forensic cases, evidence concerning the search and recovery function is often as important as the recovered data itself.

— Some tools exclusively employed by a minority of computer forensics examiners are little more than basic single-function DOS disk utilities that, when combined as a nonintegrated suite, are manipulated to perform computer forensic applications. This process has 3 fundamental problems:

1. Results from the examiners' search and recovery process are often subjective, incomplete, and variant.

2. The data restoration process can improperly alter the evidence on the evidentiary image copy or provide a visual output that is an incomplete and inaccurate reflection of the data contained on the target media.

3. Lack of integration of all essential forensic functions within the single software application presents potential challenges to the authenticity of the processed computer evidence.

— Computer forensics software should provide an objective, automated search and a data restoration process that facilitates consistency and accuracy.

— Results from search and recovery procedures that use DOS utilities vary significantly depending on the type and sequence of the nonintegrated utilities used, the amount of media to be searched, and the examiner's skill, biases, and available time.

— Each piece of acquired media must be searched separately, using the same tedious and time-consuming protocol for each hard drive, floppy drive, compact disk, and other media.

— Windows Explorer corrupts the data by altering file date stamps, temporary files, and other transient information. Better practice requires specially designed Windows-based computer forensic software that uses a noninvasive and largely automated search process.

EXPERT WITNESS TESTIMONY

— Many courts outside the United States use a high threshold to determine who is qualified to provide expert testimony regarding a technical subject.

— Threshold under Rule 702:

1. The computer forensics expert must be shown to have

"knowledge, skills, experience, training, or education" regarding the subject matter involved.

2. Trained computer forensic experts qualify as experts in US courts.

3. Prosecutors often opt not to offer the examiner as an expert, especially when records can be authenticated under Federal Rule of Evidence 901(b)(9) or a corresponding state statute or when the examiner can serve as a percipient witness, presenting objective and empirical findings of the investigation.

4. This approach tends to be more common in many state courts.

— A computer forensics examiner is commonly asked to interpret the recovered data.

Direct Examination

Pretrial Evidentiary Hearing

— If any challenge is raised to the qualifications of the computer examiner or the foundation of the evidence concerning the tools or methods used in the investigation, prosecutors prefer to address such objections outside the presence of a jury through a hearing under Federal Rule of Evidence 702, Rule 104, or *Daubert*.

— Judges are typically more receptive to technical evidence.

— This approach avoids presenting complex testimony on contested technical issues before a jury by resolving such foundational issues in a separate hearing beforehand.

Presentation of Computer Evidence

— Many prosecutors maintain that testimony concerning computer evidence should be as simple and straightforward as possible.

— Burdening the jury with overly technical information could be counterproductive and may open the door to areas of cross-examination the court would normally have disallowed.

— When seeking to establish a defendant's state of mind by presenting an electronic audit trail or connecting file date stamps, the ability to display a visual output showing various file attributes and other metadata has advantages for the advocate of such evidence.

1. The best software packages display all physical and logical data contained on the target drive, while showing the context of such files by displaying file metadata and other means.

2. When providing testimony, many examiners present evidence through screenshots in a PowerPoint presentation format or take the cloning software with them into court for a live demonstration.

BEST EVIDENCE RULE

— Doctrine or evidentiary law in the United States and Canada require that, absent some exceptions, the original of a written document or file must be admitted to prove its contents.

— Significant questions arise when applying this evidentiary doctrine to computer data.

1. How to present computer evidence at trial.

2. What constitutes a valid image of a computer drive.

3. What constitutes data compression.

"ORIGINAL" ELECTRONIC EVIDENCE

— The Federal Rules of Evidence state: "[if] data are stored in a computer or similar device, any printout or other output readable by sight, shown to reflect the data accurately is an 'original.'" Under this rule and similar rules in state jurisdictions, multiple or even an infinite number of copies of electronic files may each constitute an "original."

— The operative language is "accurate reflection."

— Bit-stream copy of a graphical image file does not provide a completely accurate "printout or other output readable by sight" unless Windows-supported forensic tools or other viewers are used non-invasively to create an accurate visual output of the recovered data, without changing any data.

— If a computer file is compressed, encrypted, and transmitted as an e-mail attachment (thereby sending a copy of that decrypted, compressed file in a different file format and even divided into many packets), and then received, decompressed, decrypted, and opened, the file in the recipient's possession would be another "original." Printing that file converts it to another file format. However, as long as the printout is an accurate reflection of the original data, it is irrelevant what the operating system or network does to that file during the printing process.

— Best Evidence Rule raised in the context of an entire drive image and an individual file:

1. When computer evidence is collected from a business, a drive image copy is often the only "original" available to the examiner, since the company often requires immediate return of the original drives to remain in business.

2. Although there is strong legal support for a drive image copy satisfying the Best Evidence Rule, it is advisable to retain physical custody of the seized drive whenever possible.

3. An ideal compromise is to retain custody of the original drives while providing restored or cloned drives to the business.

EnCase Tools

— The central component of EnCase methodology is the Evidence File, which contains the forensic bit-stream image backup made from a seized piece of computer media.

— The Evidence File consists of 3 basic parts: the file header, checksums, and data blocks. They work together to provide a secure and self-checking "exact snapshot" of the computer disk at the time of analysis.

Evidence File Format

— The EnCase process begins by creating a complete physical bit-stream forensic image of a target drive in a completely noninvasive manner.

— Except for floppy disks and CD-ROMs, evidence is acquired by the software in a DOS or Windows environment in which a specially designed, hardware write-blocking device is used.

— The acquired bit-stream forensic image is mounted as a read-only "virtual drive" from which EnCase reconstructs the file structure by reading the logical data in the bit-stream image.

— Every byte of the Evidence File is verified using a 32-bit Cyclical Redundancy Check (CRC) generated concurrent to acquisition.

— An MD5 hash is calculated for all the data contained in the evidentiary bit-stream forensic image.

— Throughout the examination process, EnCase verifies the integrity of the evidence by recalculating the CRC and MD5 hash values and comparing them with the values recorded at the time of acquisition.

— The Case Info header contains important information about the case created at the time of the file's acquisition, including:

1.   The system time, actual date, and time of acquisition.

2.   Examiner name.

3.   Notes regarding the acquisition, including case or search warrant identification numbers.

4.   Any password entered by the examiner before the acquisition of the computer evidence.

— There is no "backdoor" to the password protection.

— The information contained in the Case Info file header, with the exception of the examiner password, is documented in an integrated written reporting feature. The Case Info file header is authenticated with a separate CRC, thereby making it impossible to alter the file without registering a verification error.

Chain-of-Custody Documentation

— EnCase has documented chain-of-custody information generated at the time of acquisition and continually self-verified thereafter. EnCase reports a verification error if the Case Info file is tampered with or altered.

JURY SELECTION

Voir dire. Effective examination to determine if the juror is competent.

The Underlying Crime

— A case may involve computers, but it is above all a child abuse case and must address all traditional components of such a case.

— In luring cases, ask whether the potential juror has children or grandchildren, if those children use the Internet, and what type of supervision is provided during those sessions.

— Investigate possible stereotypes surrounding offenders.

1. In online luring cases, when the victim is teenaged and may have some emotional difficulties testifying, make the jury aware that the victim is an older child and mention any problematic issues (recantation, behavioral troubles of the victim) as early in the process as possible.

2. If the victim is a boy, bring that out immediately because many jurors assume the victim is a girl.

3. If the facts of the crime indicate the child was compliant, question jurors about how they feel about this and make them understand that this is not a defense. Laws exist to protect children from adults and from themselves.

4. In child pornography cases, explore jurors' attitudes toward child pornography and adult pornography.

   A. Inquire what, if any, media coverage of child pornography or CSE in general potential jurors have been exposed to and how they feel about the issue.

   B. Inform the jury that child pornography is not constitutionally protected.

Computers and Computer Evidence

— Deal with potential jurors' exposure to and comfort with computers.

— Ask whether the juror has ever used a computer, where, how often, and for what purposes.

— Ask if the potential juror accesses the Internet, how often, and for what purposes.

— Assess the juror's ability to listen to and understand computer evidence and a forensic examiner's testimony.

— Underplay the technical nature of the case to maximize jurors' comfort level at the beginning of the trial.

GOVERNMENT REGULATION OF THE INTERNET

— Most jurors give broad theoretical support to concepts behind the First Amendment.

— Make certain jurors understand that these free speech interests must be counterbalanced against the government's compelling interest in protecting children and prohibiting crime.

— Clarify that not all Internet speech is protected.

— Make certain jurors understand that prohibiting child pornography is not the same as regulating constitutionally protected free speech.

DIFFUSING POTENTIAL DEFENSES

— *Attack on the police and their investigatory methods.* Examine the potential bias against undercover, proactive sting tactics.

1. Check the comfort level of the juror by making it clear that these methods are legal and are used to put officers in harm's way and block an offender from successfully targeting children.

2. Address the fact that there is no real victim in a luring case. However, the fact that the police took on the persona of a child does not mean that a crime did not occur.

3. In a pornography case, clarify that though the image of a child was sent to a police officer rather than someone else, it does not mean the defendant is innocent.

— *Mistaken identity.* Describe the types of evidence or factors a potential juror would look for in determining the identity in any case and then in a computer-facilitated case.

— *Necessary element of intent not present.* Help jurors see through types of untrue defense.

— *First Amendment or Privilege Defense.* Defendants admit to the possession of child pornography but claim they possess it in furtherance of activity protected by the Constitution or for a legally viable reason (reporter working on a story, medical practitioner who needs it for a book about child sexual abuse, etc).

1. If the defendant had a legitimate purpose for the contraband and the law allows for such possession, the state may still contend that the defendant was using it for purposes outside the prescribed exemption.

2. Inquire how the juror would go about deciding if the defendant had a legitimate purpose.

— *Virtual child pornography defense.* Prosecution must now prove that the image of child pornography is of a real child.

1. It is not necessary to prove the identity of the child.

2. Question jurors regarding their awareness of the case of *Ashcroft v Free Speech Coalition* (2002) and their understanding of it.

3. If the defense is planning to call an expert to testify that the images are completely computer generated and the state will call its own expert to refute this claim, ask jurors how they would handle conflicting reports and expert testimony in general.

— *Conducting voir dire.* Prosecutors must consider their own personality and courtroom persona style.

1. See this as an opportunity to educate jurors and gauge potential jurors' attitudes and beliefs about key aspects of cases.

2. The best voir dire incorporates personal style with specific cases, potential jurors, judge, local rules and practices, and other external factors.

MEETING UNTRUE DEFENSES
MISTAKEN IDENTITY
— Keep in mind conventional investigative techniques common to all cases, such as surveillance of suspect's home, observing who enters and leaves, talking to neighbors, and interviewing the suspect.

— Perform recorded pretext telephone calls to determine who is at the computer terminal at any particular time and if anyone else has access.

— Review sign-on logs or engage in surveillance and video monitoring to help identify the suspect.

— Meet the suspect face-to-face in a public location in a sting operation.

— Consider the use of no-knock warrants.

— Perform forensic examinations to verify or refute suspects' claims that they gave someone else their user/screen names and passwords to go online.

DEFEATING HACKER/INTRUSION DEFENSES

— Use general knowledge of computer operating systems and other computer basics to overcome the defense.

— Forensic examiners can detect the Trojan-horse type programs used by hackers to remotely program and control a computer.

PROOF OF REAL VERSUS COMPUTER-GENERATED IMAGES AND AGE ISSUES

— Prove the child is real using:

1. Testimony of the child or someone who knows the child.

2. An expert in the history of child pornography to testify that the computer image the defendant distributed came from a magazine printed in an era when individuals could not yet create or alter such an image on a personal computer.

3. A computer graphics expert to evaluate the pixels or shading differences in an image to determine if the image was altered and testify concerning morphing software.

— The government does not need to prove exact age but must prove that the person depicted is not an adult.

— Prove age via:

1. Testimony of the minor or someone who knows the minor.

2. An expert such as a pediatrician, who offers an opinion as to the age of the depicted person (see Chapter 7, Medical Issues).

3. A lay witness who gives an opinion of the age.

4. Permitting the jury to decide and to draw its own conclusions from the evidence presented.

— May need to prove the defendant specifically sought images of children by reviewing their computer history.

LACK OF INTENT

— In an entrapment defense, the crime must be induced or encouraged by the government agents.

— Key concepts are inducement and predisposition.

1. *Inducement.* Government agents induced offender to commit the crime. Can include pressure, assurance the person is doing nothing wrong, persuasion, fraudulent representations, threats, coercive tactics, harassment, promises of reward, or pleas based on need, sympathy, or friendship. Was defendant eager or reluctant to participate in the alleged criminal conduct?

2. *Predisposition.* Analyze (a) the character or reputation of the defendant, (b) whether the suggestion of criminal activity was originally made by government, (c) whether the defendant was engaged in criminal activity for profit, (d) whether the defendant evidenced reluctance to commit offense, overcome by government persuasion, and (e) the nature of the inducement or persuasion offered.

— In response to this defense, the government may want to propose an instruction to reduce the likelihood of jury nullification when the jury acquits the defendant in disregard of the judge's instructions and contrary to the jury's finding of fact because they have sympathy for the defendant or regard the law unfavorably.

— The advantage of claiming entrapment is that it may allow character evidence, proof of prior crimes or bad acts, hearsay, etc, to be admitted when these would have otherwise not been admissible.

INTERNET ADDICTION

— Currently, there are no published cases where Internet addiction has been presented successfully as a substantive defense in a criminal case.

— No causal relationships have as yet been established between specific addictive behaviors and their cause.

— Addiction is irrelevant to the issue: if the addiction is to the Internet, it does not explain why defendant obtained, maintained, or organized child pornography files.

ACCIDENT

— This defense is refuted by complete forensic examination of the suspect's computer to reveal Web sites visited and Usenet newsgroups subscribed to.

— Appeal to jurors to consider how many times they have ever experienced computers generating new data rather than losing or destroying existing data. Generally, accidents destroy data rather than create it.

DELETED COMPUTER IMAGES

— Defendants can claim they did not know they possessed child pornography because they thought they had deleted it.

— The ability to destroy is evidence of control. The destruction of contraband does not lead to conclusion that one never possessed it but rather that one did.

MERE VIEWING

— Even when the defendant does not personally download images, the defendant still has control over them and is the possessor.

FIRST AMENDMENT

— Some jurisdictions allow for certain categories of individuals to possess child pornography pursuant to statute.

— Test is twofold. Do they have a professional use for the material? Were they using it professionally?

— There are no other recognized exceptions.

REFERENCES

Daubert v Merrell Dow Pharmaceuticals, Inc, 509 US 579,592-594, 113 S Ct 2786, 125 L Ed 2d 469 (1993).

Fed R Evidence 702.

Fed R Evidence 901.

Frye v United States, 293 F 1013 (DC Cir 1923).

Lanning K. *Child Molesters: A Behavioral Analysis for Law Enforcement Officers Investigating the Sexual Exploitation of Children by Acquaintance Molesters.* 4th ed. Arlington, Va: National Center for Missing & Exploited Children; September 2001.

United States v Anderson, 154 F3d 1225 (10th Cir 1998).

United States v Anderson, 187 F3d 649 (unpublished) (1999).

United States v Garcia, 983 F2d 1160 (1st Cir 1993).

United States v Grimes, 244 F3d 375 (5th Cir 2001).

United States v Hill, 322 F Sup 2d 1081 (CD Cal 2004).

United States v Horn, 187 F3d 781 (8th Cir 1999).

United States v Hotal, 143 F3d 1223 (9th Cir 1998).

United States v Lamb, 945 F Supp 441 (NDNY 1996).

United States v Layne, 43 F3d 127 (5th Cir 1995).

United States v Loy, 191 F3d 360 (3rd Cir 1999).

United States v Pitts, 6 F3d 1366 (9th Cir 1993).

United States v Ricciardelli, 998 F2d 8 (1st Cir 1993).

United States v Rowland, 145 F3d 1194 (10th Cir 1998).

United States v Simpson, 152 F3d 1241 (10th Cir 1998).

Chapter 15

SUPPORT SERVICES FOR PROSTITUTED CHILDREN

Mary P. Alexander, MA, LPC
Elena Azaola, PhD
Richard J. Estes, DSW, ACSW
Fadi Barakat Fadel
Nicole G. Ives, MSW, PhD (Candidate)
Nancy D. Kellogg, MD
Mary Anne Layden, PhD
Daniel J. Sheridan, PhD, RN, FAAN
Linnea W. Smith, MD
Phyllis Thompson, LCSW
Dawn Van Pelt, BSN, RN

SCOPE OF THE PROBLEM

— Services must address the issues faced by prostituted youths.

1. Childhood sexual abuse (Farley & Barkan, 1998)

2. Incest

3. Use of physical force during their first intercourse, rape, or multiple rapes (James & Meyerding, 1977)

— Treatment is generally offered in a fragmented fashion that reflects the outcomes of prostitution and victimization rather than the underlying causes.

— Short-term therapy is available, but it rarely addresses sexual victimization.

— Victims are reluctant to expose abuse and eager to avoid treatment.

BARRIERS TO LEAVING PROSTITUTION
— Traumatic bonding

1. This type of bonding is characterized by intermittent, unpredictable abuse and power imbalances that can produce powerful emotional attachments, even in new relationships.

2. A victim is isolated from a caring family or friends, intermittently abused, and then goes through a period of improved relationship with the abuser that feeds the victim's fantasy of being loved (Dutton & Painter, 1993).

— Victims have learned to mistrust adults.

— Victims suffer severely eroded self-esteem.

— To stay off the streets, victims need support from someone who has experienced what they have experienced.

— Victims also need a support system that meets the needs of their new lifestyle.

— The most commonly used harm-reduction methods do not address the complex issues children face.

EXITING THE SEX TRADE LIFESTYLE
— Some victims are constantly looking for ways out, but many stumble on an opportunity to exit.

— Specific reasons are generally cited, but these vary from case to case and include unforeseen circumstances such as pregnancy, drug overdose, violence, and rape.

— Even after deciding to exit, victims struggle and fall back into the trade because existing crisis intervention services have gaps such as:

1. Insufficient outreach personnel

2. Insufficient detoxification and treatment beds for youths

3. Lack of residential mental health facilities

4.   Lack of safe, supportive, residential environments specifically designed for youths

— Healing begins when these children accept that they are victims of abuse and exploitation and did not choose their lifestyle. They need to forgive themselves.

SUCCESSFUL EXITING AND HEALING
— Must address:

1.   Housing

2.   Economic opportunities and skills development

3.   Ability to adopt healthy behaviors

— Must involve:

1.   Access to quality services and peer support

2.   Strong and meaningful support from individuals and community services

STAGES OF EXITING AND HEALING GROUPS
— *Inclusion.* Participants become informed and oriented to the group, the members, and the therapist/facilitator.

— *Conflict.* Participants face the reality of the situation and see the task ahead as enormous. This is the most difficult stage; it is characterized by frustration, ambiguity, and anxiety and has a high rate of relapse.

— *Resolution.* Reconciliation between reality and the expectations of members, the organization as a whole, and outside players occurs. The group begins to examine goals in the light of the time limits, tasks to be accomplished, restrictions of the situation, and skills available. What happens at this time influences the depth, quality, and success of the exiting and healing process.

— *Production.* This is the most productive stage, with attention focused on the task with a renewed anticipation, hope, and positive feeling of eagerness to participate.

— *Termination.* The process reaches its end, and the task is completed or the time allotted has run out (Kass, 1996).

1. If the task is completed or the group has worked through the issues of interdependence and cohesion, enormous benefits result.

2. If the group terminates before this is accomplished, negative outcomes can occur.

GOVERNMENTAL PROGRAMS

— Prevention, prosecution, and protection are central aspects of the US campaign against the commercial sexual exploitation of children (CSEC).

— Program goals:

1. Increase public awareness about the existence of CSEC.

2. Increase societal intolerance for all forms of CSEC.

3. Initiate cooperative law enforcement activities among Canada, Mexico, and United States for dealing with cross-border and regional aspects of CSEC.

4. Create a more comprehensive system of local, state, and federal protection for child victims of commercial sexual exploitation and their families.

— Children involved in prostitution, survival sex, and other types of sex-for-money exchanges have received comparatively modest attention from the central government because:

1. Prostitution at any age in the United States is defined principally as a local rather than a federal issue, so local law enforcement officials handle the cases.

2. Prostitution of juveniles is not perceived as widespread or potentially harmful compared to child pornography.

3. Law enforcement and human service resources that handle juvenile prostitution are complex, expensive, and currently allocated to other policing functions.

— New laws and stronger existing laws increase the age of sexual consent for juveniles, impose stringent age disparity penalties on adults convicted of engaging in sexual relationships with juveniles, and classify sex tourism as a crime.

— Prosecutorial Remedies and Other Tools To End the Exploitation of Children Today (PROTECT) Act:

1. Makes it a crime for citizens or legal residents of the United States to engage in sexual acts with a person younger than 18 years in a foreign country.

2. Removes previous legal requirements for proof of intention to engage in such acts before travel.

3. Strengthens sentencing guideline provisions for offenders.

4. Adds provisions requiring mandatory minimum sentencing requirements to deal with repeat offenders.

5. Provides law enforcement personnel with new tools for dealing with child prostitution, trafficking, and child pornography.

HEALTHCARE SETTINGS

— Victims may enter a setting with medical or psychiatric problems related to victimization. Generally they seek services only after physical or psychological symptoms become extreme.

— Protocols for victims of physical and sexual abuse:

1. Police and child protective services (CPS) agencies should be notified.

2. CPS is responsible for developing and enforcing immediate safety plans, follow-up care, and support services, including visits to hospital emergency rooms, community child abuse centers, and specialized outpatient settings.

AMBULATORY CARE CLINICS

Victims of juvenile prostitution may use these facilities while they continue to reside with their families, who may or may not be aware of situation.

EMERGENCY CARE FACILITIES

— Victims may be brought by law enforcement personnel if the victimization is witnessed or if they appear to have significant health problems.

— When children and adolescents do not come voluntarily for medical care, the need for a comprehensive assessment of risky behaviors is clear.

— Note victims' emotional state:

1. Emotional state may range from inconsolable crying and shaking to tightly controlled response.

2. Note any incongruent affect or combative or intoxicated victims who may claim to be unable to remember what happened before they woke up with various injuries or found their clothes gone or in disarray.

3. Victims often deflect questions about abusive experiences to avoid discovery and having to file a child abuse report with authorities.

— Emergency care personnel must remain calm and reassuring, maintain control of their emotions, give choices to victims, and provide developmentally appropriate information.

MENTAL HEALTH CLINICS

— Prostituted youths are at increased risk for depression, suicide, post-traumatic stress disorder (PTSD), and neuroses (Gibson-Ainyetteet et al, 1988; Seng, 1989; Yates et al, 1991).

— They may come for care of acute overdoses or other forms of self-injury.

— Personnel must respond appropriately and know about available community resources.

JUVENILE DETENTION FACILITIES

— Victims are often seen after arrest for distribution or possession of an illegal substance, public intoxication, running away, prostitution, burglary, possession of an illegal weapon, aggravated assault, or aggravated robbery.

— Detained children commonly demonstrate a lack of trust or co-oper-ation and anger.

INITIAL ASSESSMENT OF VICTIM
See Chapter 7, Medical Issues.

PSYCHIATRIC ASSESSMENT
— Violent, combative behavior directed against others or themselves is common.

— Most obvious diagnostic presentations are substance-related disorders, dissociative disorders, impulse control, and antisocial personality traits, as well as most or all of the Axis IV psychosocial and environmental problems in *Diagnostic and Statistical Manual of Mental Disorders*, 4th ed.

— Employ emergency restraint and sedation for combative youths.

— Make an immediate referral to a psychiatrist for those who are homicidal or suicidal.

— Be aware that some will develop psychoses and need immediate psychiatric assessment.

— Remain calm, unrushed, and caring in order to obtain the information necessary for making an appropriate assessment.

Major Depressive Disorders and Posttraumatic Stress Disorder
— Symptoms include hypervigilance, difficulty concentrating, exaggerated startle response, rage, dissociation, denial, autonomic arousal, insomnia, nightmares, psychic numbing, and recurrent or intrusive memories of the abuse.

— Victims are often self-medicating with drugs or alcohol.

— By the time they are diagnosed, children and adolescents have developed successful survival skills so they can avoid disclosing the abuse or recalling their traumatic events for months or years.

— The first time these victims are drug free and sober may be during incarceration, thus detention and secured placement may provide the best opportunities for therapeutic interventions.

1. The pain in their lives may begin to erode the walls they have erected.

2. First stage is addressing the trauma, decreasing anxiety, and treating depression.

3. Better long-term results occur when substance-related disorders are identified, acknowledged as significant, and properly treated.

— Obsessive-compulsive behaviors are often missed if a clinician spends only short amounts of time with a child and does not interview family members. Such behaviors represent victims' efforts to control insignificant events in their lives in order to counter the barrage of destructive and demoralizing events they cannot control.

DEVELOPMENTAL, BEHAVIORAL, AND EMOTIONAL ASSESSMENT

— A significant portion of prostituted youths have physical, cognitive, emotional, and social delays.

— Delays may be related to premature birth, maternal substance abuse, or other maternal behaviors that harmed the fetus.

— Cognitive deficits and learning disabilities may reflect either exposure to drugs in utero or chronic substance abuse during childhood or adolescence.

— The most common conditions include attention-deficit/hyperactivity disorder and conduct disorder.

Attention-Deficit/Hyperactivity Disorder

— Persistent pattern of inattention and/or hyperactivity/impulsivity is found more often and to a more severe degree than in persons at comparable developmental levels (American Psychiatric Association [APA], 1994).

— Common symptoms include inability to concentrate, distractibility, avoidance, and hyperactivity.

— Also show symptoms similar to those of PTSD.

— Explore possibilities of previous trauma, onset, and duration of symptoms to differentiate from PTSD.

Conduct Disorder
— Conduct disorder:

1. Is a persistent pattern of behaviors that violate the basic rights of others and/or the accepted societal norms or rules.

2. May include aggression toward animals, people, or property; deceitful behavior; or theft (APA, 1994).

3. Reflects chaotic home environment and contributes to school difficulties during preadolescence, truancy, and dropping out in adolescence.

4. Is exacerbated when child is in a closed or secured facility; many need placement in isolation.

— Assess language and cognitive skills of victims and structure interview questions and therapy plans accordingly.

— A claim not to have a behavioral or emotional problem may be a reflection of acceptance and accommodation of victimization or a barrier created to avoid potential friends.

INTERMEDIATE AND LONG-TERM COMMUNITY AND MENTAL HEALTH SUPPORT
— Success depends on willingness of a victim to undergo therapy, support from a parent or custodial agency, and the availability of shelters and resources, educational opportunities, and effective therapeutic programs in clinical and neighborhood settings.

— Homeless prostituted youths are unlikely to engage in therapy unless placed in prisons or lock-up treatment facilities where such treatment is mandatory.

— Community and school clinics:

1. These clinics may be the most effective means of identifying youths at risk for prostitution (Rickel & Hendren, 1992).

2. Clinics are more accessible to street youths, but long-term use is rare.

3. Some youths may be denied access to shelter services if they have no identification (Unger et al, 1998).

4. Lesbian, gay, bisexual, and transgender youths are often subjected to abuse from other homeless children and adolescents in shelters (Hofstede, 1999).

5. Clinics must focus on accessibility, safety, constructive survival skills, and providing basic resources and childcare along with medical, legal, and therapeutic services.

6. Immediate needs of street youths include food and shelter; education about substance use dangers, gangs, and human immunodeficiency virus-risk behaviors; and assistance with transition from street life to stable living and work environments (Unger et al, 1998; Yates et al, 1991).

7. As mandated reporters, service providers must report allegations of child abuse to law enforcement and/or CPS.

8. Community programs must also address routine and systemic assessments of the relationship between neighborhood opportunities and recruitment into prostitution (Longres, 1991), incorporating:

   A. Self-help and social support networks between concerned or threatened families and youths.

   B. Community education on prostitution, recruitment into prostitution, pornography, and gang involvement.

   C. Community watches and efforts to remove prostitution from identified residential areas.

   D. Enhancement of regional legitimate economic opportunities for adults and youths engaged in prostitution (Longres, 1991).

9. Resources include supportive parents of adjudicated youths.

— Younger victims benefit most from therapy with specialized sexual assault therapists.

GOALS OF LONG-TERM THERAPY
— Goals vary with age but generally are:

1. Reduce high-risk health behaviors.

2. Enhance decision-making skills.

3. Address gender and other identity issues.

4. Establish a positive support system.

5. Instill a sense of hope and positive outlook toward the future.

6. Identify a permanent safe harbor.

— Most effective long-term therapy:

1. Effective therapy begins with a 9- or 12-month stay in a secured environment. This step ensures safety and cessation of substance abuse, runaway behavior, and prostitution while addressing issues that led to the deleterious lifestyle.

2. Effective therapy also provides for good physical health and emotional stability as the foundation for therapeutic intervention. Juveniles provided with the needed medical care, psychiatric care, medications, exercise, relaxation skills, and monitoring begin to feel better physically and become motivated to maintain the healthier self.

3. Individual counseling:

   A. In weekly sessions, youths can establish trusting relationship with responsible adult.

   B. Therapist models appropriate adult-child boundaries.

   C. Individual sessions provide an opportunity to address difficult issues in safe environment.

   D. Victims should have some input into development of treatment plan.

   E. Therapist must incorporate strategies to enhance learning skills to decrease anxiety, experience small successes, detach from unhealthy relationships, and obtain ideas, suggestions, and opportunities to establish a new or different healthy support network.

   F. Counseling may facilitate cognitive restructuring, correct unhealthy cognitive distortions, provide clarification for confusing issues, teach relaxation techniques, and help the child or adolescent develop healthy relationships.

G. Treatment plan becomes tool for measuring progress, helping therapist recognize successes and patterns of self-defeating thoughts or behaviors.

H. Adjust approach to reinforce positive attitudes and behavior; address thinking errors and poor judgment, rationalizations, or unhealthy avoidant behaviors.

I. Gather pertinent family information and specific topics to address in later group sessions.

4. Group sessions:

A. Provide vital peer feedback for inappropriate behaviors. Juveniles are often more receptive when confronted by peers about destructive behaviors, poor decisions, and life-threatening behaviors.

B. Common themes include substance abuse, lack of trust, promiscuous sexual behavior, family violence, antisocial behaviors, and poor problem-solving skills.

C. Therapist guides and monitors topics, maintains clear boundaries, and ensures a safe environment.

D. Commonalities of family dynamics and worldviews facilitate acceptance and participation in the group support system.

E. Long-term group therapy provides a temporary support system and promotes the development of the self-esteem and self-reliance needed to reenter society and establish healthy, more permanent support systems.

5. Family therapy:

A. If placement back into the home is possible, begin family therapy about 3 months before the reunification.

B. Encourage all family members in the home to participate.

C. Encourage and positively reinforce the attendance of the primary caregiver at weekly family sessions.

D. If family members do not attend, help victims understand and cope with unsupportive family members.

6. If victims cannot return home, enroll them in a general equivalency diploma program and job training.

    A. Obtaining financial, educational, and emotional independence is critical to positive outcomes.

    B. Goal is to provide proper tools, self-confidence, and ego strength needed to live independently and have hope for a positive future.

7. Placement in a foster home, relative's home, or with alternative caregiver: Provide therapeutic follow-up care 2 to 4 times per month for 6 months.

8. When a crisis occurs or victims desire more frequent contact, provide such services.

9. Also provide legal and therapeutic support for juveniles who will be called to testify in legal proceedings against abusers or pimps.

10. Be aware that during reunification, adolescents are at risk for reassociating with their previous peer group and beginning problematic behaviors again.

SPECIAL ISSUES FOR BOYS

— More boys report engaging in prostitution for pleasure and money than girls and often identify themselves as hustlers rather than as prostituted.

— Between 25% and 35% identify themselves as gay, bisexual, or transgender/transsexual.

— Prostituted boys and men often have gender identity conflict (Boyer, 1989; Savin-Williams, 1994). The stigma associated with homosexuality hinders their reports of abuse and they sometimes come to identify themselves with the aggressors and become pimps (Boyer, 1989).

— Family members may further alienate victims because of sexual orientation issues (Savin-Williams, 1994).

SAFETY ISSUES
— Because family members are often perpetrators or are unable to support and protect their children, identifying a permanent safe place for prostituted children can be problematic.

— Shelters or foster homes serve for short-term placements; adoption or reunification with family members provide longer-term solutions when appropriate.

SPECIFIC THERAPEUTIC APPROACHES
VISUAL CUES
Because children and adolescents are concrete thinkers and visually oriented, they need concrete cues to demonstrate abstract concepts and enhance their ability to retain and understand such concepts.

FAMILY HISTORY AND FAMILY GENOGRAMS
— Characteristics of families of prostituted youths. See Chapter 2, Victims and Offenders.

— A genogram is obtained in third or fourth counseling session and consists of information about the family that reveals patterns and behaviors. It is used to establish relationships and ask questions that may lead children to spontaneously share details about their family and childhood experiences.

LONG-TERM PROGNOSIS
— Program goals include short-term recovery from victimization and long-term resiliency.

— Highly developed cognitive skills may lead to academic success and a sense of competence or more effective coping strategies in abused children (Cicchetti et al, 1993).

— A sense of self-worth helps protect against depression (Moran & Echenrode, 1992) and/or moderates the effects of ongoing negative messages (Cicchetti et al, 1993).

— Resiliency:

1. Resiliency is associated with an internal locus of control for good events. Individuals understand that they have power and control over certain aspects of their lives.

2. Victims are healthier when they realize that good things happen to them because of who they are or what they do, not because of luck or factors out of their control.

3. External attribution of blame with regard to sexually abusive experiences appears to enhance resiliency (Valentine & Feinauer, 1993).

4. Spirituality, having a sense of purpose in life, and feelings of self-worth in spite of abusive experiences are facilitated by involvement in a religious support group, which also serves as an external support system (Heller et al, 1999).

5. Ego control (one's level of susceptibility or vulnerability to the environment) is associated with resiliency in maltreated children (Cicchetti et al, 1993).

6. Characteristics of resiliency include reflectiveness, persistence, attentiveness, dependability, and relaxation, with greater awareness and avoidance of risk factors for maltreatment (Cicchetti et al, 1993).

7. Family cohesions (presence of sensitive, consistent, and safe caregiving environment) (Heller et al, 1999) are related to resiliency after maltreatment (Egeland et al, 1993; Romans et al, 1995; Toth & Cicchetti, 1996).

8. Extrafamilial support includes school involvement, extracurricular activities or hobbies, and religious group involvement, all related to resiliency (Egeland et al, 1993; Herrenkohl et al, 1994).

9. Positive experiences in extrafamilial or intrafamilial support systems enhance self-esteem and feelings of self-worth.

SCREENING PROGRAMS

— Abuse Assessment Screen (Soeken et al, 1998) (**Table 15-1**):

1. Used effectively with adult and adolescent girls.

2. Consists of 2 to 6 questions.

3. Screens for physical, sexual, emotional, and psychological abuse, including fear of harm.

— Screening should be conducted in a private setting.

— Preface all screening efforts with a global statement that you, as a concerned practitioner, routinely screen all patients for violence because it is so common in society. Do not promise complete confidentiality because mandatory reporting statutes may require notification of the police and/or CPS.

— Assure patients they can return to the healthcare setting any time for any reason.

Table 15-1. Abuse Assessment Screen

1. When you and your partner argue, are you ever afraid of him?

2. When you and your partner argue, do you think he is trying to emotionally hurt (abuse) you?

3. Does your partner try to control you? Who you see? Where you can go?

4. Has your partner ever hit, slapped, pushed, kicked, or otherwise physically hurt you?

5. Since you have been pregnant (or when you were pregnant), has your partner (or anyone) hit, slapped, pushed, kicked, or otherwise physically hurt you?

6. Has your partner (or anyone) forced you into sex when you did not want to participate?

With any and every answer of "yes," thank the patient for sharing the information, then ask for an example and when it last occurred.

Adapted with permission from Daniel J. Sheridan.

SAFETY PLANNING

— Creative safety planning should provide victims options for safely leaving relationships marked by interpersonal violence.

— Have a team approach to safety planning, including on-site social workers, forensically trained nurses, and community-based advocates.

— Provide victims with access to a telephone in a private setting and connect the victim to a 24-hour helpline expert.

— Failure to screen, document, and refer places the provider at a liability risk and at risk for noncompliance with federal healthcare regulatory guidelines such as those established by the Joint Commission on the Accreditation of Healthcare Organizations and the Centers for Medicaid and Medicare Services.

PRINCIPLES OF GOOD PRACTICE

See **Table 15-2**.

Table 15-2. Principles of Good Practice	
PRINCIPLE	DESCRIPTION
Meaningful and visible decision making of experiential children and youths	The victim must play a meaningful and visible decision-making role in developing efforts, especially in the participation system itself.
Realistic participation	All aspects of participation must be realistic and appropriate to the circumstances.
Capacity-building	Those who personally experienced exploitation are supported through creation and delivery of services.
Recognition of expertise	Recognize the children and youths are the only experts on CSEC; they should be paid for their expertise and considered seriously for employment opportunities.

(continued)

Table 15-2. *(continued)*

PRINCIPLE	DESCRIPTION
Meaningful exchange	Include in efforts to address CSEC the capacity or opportunity for meaningful exchange among the partners.
Safe, voluntary, and confidential participation	Safety is the primary concern. Respecting the victims' anonymity and explicitly acknowledging their confidentiality facilitates voluntary involvement.
Self-help	Acknowledge the value of youths' ability to help themselves and each other. Create opportunities to gather together and talk with each other with no fear of repercussion.
Accountability	Young people must be able to play a role in monitoring and evaluating the actions taken by government and the community in addressing CSEC.
Flexibility	The meeting times, styles, and locations must reflect the needs of the victims.
Commitment to outcomes	Everyone involved must be committed to change.
Long-term vision	The process takes time and must include focusing on underlying factors and not merely surface symptoms.
Meeting people where they are	Physically go to locations where youths feel safe and comfortable or find imaginative ways to accommodate the needs of youths so the process belongs to them.

REFERENCES

American Psychiatric Association (APA). *Diagnostic and Statistical Manual of Mental Disorders.* 4th ed. Washington, DC: APA; 1994.

Boyer D. Male prostitution and homosexual identity. *J Homosex.* 1989;17(1-2):151-184.

Cicchetti D, Rogosch ML, Holt KD. Resilience in maltreated children: processes leading to adaptive outcome. *Dev Psychopathol.* 1993;5: 626-647.

Dutton DG, Painter SL. Traumatic bonding: the development of emotional attachments in battered women and other relationships of intermittent abuse. *Victimology.* 1981;1:139-155.

Egeland B, Carlson E, Sroufe LA. Resilience as process. *Dev Psychopathol.* 1993;5:517-528.

Farley M, Barkan H. Prostitution, violence, and posttraumatic stress disorder. *Women Health.* 1998;27:37-49.

Gibson-Ainyette I, Templer DI, Brown R, Veaco L. Adolescent female prostitutes. *Arch Sex Behav.* 1988;17(5):431-438.

Heller SS, Larrieu JA, D'Imperio R, Boris NW. Research on resilience to child maltreatment: empirical considerations. *Child Abuse Negl.* 1999;23(4):321-338.

Herrenkohl EC, Herrenkohl R, Egolf B. Resilient early school-age children from maltreating homes: outcomes in late adolescence. *Am J Orthopsychiatry.* 1994;64:301-309.

Hofstede A. The Hofstede Committee report: juvenile prostitution in Minnesota: 1999. Available at: http://www.ag.state.mn.us/consumer/PDF/hofstede.pdf. Accessed September 16, 2003.

James J, Meyerding J. Early sexual experience and prostitution. *Am J Psychiatry.* 1977;134:1381-1385.

Kass R. *Theories in Group Development.* Montreal, Canada: Concordia University; 1996.

Longres JF. An ecological study of parents of adjudicated female teenage prostitutes. *J Soc Serv Res.* 1991;14(2):113-127.

Moran PB, Eckenrode J. Protective personality characteristics among adolescent victims of maltreatment. *Child Abuse Negl.* 1992;16:743-754.

Rickel AU, Hendren MC. Aberrant sexual experiences in adolescence. In: Gullotta TP, Adams GR, Montemayor R, eds. *Adolescent Sexuality.* Newbury Park, Calif: Sage Publications; 1992:141-160. *Advances in Adolescent Development Series*; vol 5.

Romans SE, Martin JL, Anderson JC, O'Shea ML, Mullen PE. Factors that mediate between child sexual abuse and adult psychological outcome. *Psychol Med.* 1995;25:127-142.

Savin-Williams RC. Verbal and physical abuse as stressors in the lives of lesbian, gay male, and bisexual youth: associations with school problems, running away, substance abuse, prostitution, and suicide. *J Consult Clin Psychol.* 1994;62(2):261-269.

Seng MJ. Child sexual abuse and adolescent prostitution: a comparative analysis. *Adolescence.* 1989;24(95):665-675.

Soeken KL, McFarlane J, Parker B, Lominak MC. The abuse assessment screen: measuring frequency, severity, and perpetrator abuse against women. In: Campbell JC, ed. *Empowering Survivors of Abuse: Health Care for Battered Women and Their Children.* Thousand Oaks, Calif: Sage Publications; 1998:195-203.

Toth SL, Cicchetti D. Patterns of relatedness, depressive symptomatology, and perceived competence in maltreated children. *J Consult Clin Psychol.* 1996;64:32-41.

Unger JB, Simon TR, Newman TL, Montgomery SB, Kipke MD, Albornoz M. Early adolescent street youth: an overlooked population with unique problems and service needs. *J Early Adolesc.* 1998;18(4): 325-349.

Valentine L, Feinauer LL. Resilience factors associated with female survivors of childhood sexual abuse. *Am J Fam Ther.* 1993;21:216-224.

Yates GL, MacKenzie RG, Pennbridge J, Swofford A. A risk profile comparison of homeless youth involved in prostitution and homeless youth not involved. *J Adolesc Health.* 1991;12:545-548.

Chapter 16

AMBER Alert

Sharon W. Cooper, MD, FAAP

— Report of a missing child who has been abducted under certain circumstances may constitute an emergency, mandating an immediate, competent law enforcement response.

— The AMBER Alert process is initiated when a child is missing and considered to be in imminent danger.

— A coalition involving the emergency broadcast system, law enforcement agencies, and the department of transportation provide the response capability to facilitate the recovery of such abducted children.

— First, law enforcement officials verify that an authentic need exists for the alert to be initiated. A message is broadcast via radio and/or television and displayed on highway signs. This solicits the help of private citizens who search for the described motor vehicle and license plate number so law enforcement personnel can be notified as soon as possible after a sighting. The operation has resulted in numerous safe outcomes.

— Notification process:

1. Law enforcement officials help validate the degree of threat to the child.

2. Increased harm is associated with a known abductor, a history of substance abuse and/or violence, prior criminal record, or witness report of presence or possession of a weapon.

3. The local broadcast system is then notified and the appropriate range of dissemination of the information is confirmed.

— Message broadcasted includes the vehicle's description and/or license plate information whenever possible.

— Abductors often relinquish custody of the victim and turn themselves in to investigators when they realize the futility of attempt-ing to escape this coordinated community effort.

— **Table 16-1** lists the contact information for foundations and victim support services.

ROLE OF NATIONAL AMBER ALERT COORDINATOR

— Is held by Assistant Attorney General for the Office of Justice Programs.

— Is responsible for assisting state and local officials as they develop and enhance AMBER plans and promoting statewide and regional coordination among the plans. Specifically, the national coordinator:

Table 16-1. Currently Active Foundations and Victim Support Services

National Center for Missing & Exploited Children (NCMEC)
— 1-800-THE-LOST
— http://www.missingkids.com

Jacob Wetterling Foundation
— http://www.jwf.org

The Polly Klaas Foundation
— http://www.pollyklaas.org

KlaasKids Foundation
— http://www.klaaskids.org

Megan Nicole Kanka Foundation
— http://www.megannicolekankafoundation.org

The Jimmy Ryce Center for Victims of Predatory Abduction
— http://www.jimmy-ryce.org

---

1. Facilitates the AMBER network development.

2. Provides support for the development of state AMBER plans and efforts.

3. Increases efforts to eliminate geographic gaps in AMBER networks.

4. Provides regional AMBER network coordination.

5. Establishes guidance criteria to ensure an AMBER Alert.

ABDUCTION OF INFANTS

— Infant abductions are a particular concern for hospitals with birthing units or newborn nurseries. Additional risk occurs during the neonatal period of 4 weeks postpartum, when infants have been discharged to homes and home health care agencies are providing services.

— Birth announcements are often posted in newspapers or on gender-specific signs placed in front yards of homes, thereby unintentionally putting the newborn at risk for possible abduction attempts.

STRATEGY FOR AMBER COORDINATION

— National advisory group includes the US Department of Justice, US Department of Transportation, National Center for Missing and Exploited Children, television and radio broadcasters, and law enforcement personnel.

— The advisory group works to develop a strategy for support in states and communities where the system is beginning to be used.

— A major factor to consider in these cases is the nature of the community. Dynamics of urban communities differ considerably from those of rural communities regarding the nature of the crime of abduction, skill of local law enforcement officers, and caliber of transportation department support capability.

— 3 important aspects of the national strategy:

1. Assessment of current AMBER activity

    A. Determine the number of existing plans.

    B. Identify management of organization (law enforcement

agencies, state broadcasters' association, state Attorney General's office).

    C. Compare plan operations and establish clear community notification criteria for each local group.

    D. Assess each community's available technology.

2.   Creation of a coordinated AMBER network

    A. Seek to develop guidelines for criteria used to issue an AMBER Alert.

    B. Use guidelines to train local agencies about risk factors that elevate the degree of urgency in a case.

    C. Establish federal, state, and local partnerships that share the success of the AMBER Alert process.

    D. Promote technological compatibility among communication systems.

    E. Requires expert technology consultation coordination so a universal cyberspace language exists when 1 emergency notification agency communicates with another.

    F. Funding requires assistance from federal government and local partnerships.

3.   Communication of lessons learned

    A. Provide experiential learning for participants as they establish working relationships.

    B. Assist state and community officials as they develop AMBER Alert plans to avoid repeating the errors of older, more established programs.

    C. Raise public awareness of how to protect children and prevent abduction.

CHILD LURE PREVENTION

— Develop educational program for parents, children, and educators.

— Present reported abduction and sexual offense situations plus suggestions for actions the child may use to escape or avoid being victimized.

— Recognize that child abductions are often well planned.

ATTEMPTED NONFAMILY ABDUCTIONS

NATIONAL INCIDENCE STUDY OF MISSING, ABDUCTED, RUNAWAY, AND THROWNAWAY CHILDREN IN AMERICA

— Includes incidents when a nonfamily member tries to take, detain, or lure a child (Finkelhor et al, 1990).

— Most attempts are lures wherein strangers try to get the child to accompany them in their cars.

— Stereotypical kidnappings (Sedlak et al, 2002):

1. 200 to 300 occur per year.

2. Child is kept 1 night, transported 50 miles, held for ransom, or killed.

— Criteria for "missing" is that the victim is younger than 18 years and the situation falls into one of the following categories (Sedlak et al, 2002):

1. Nonfamily abduction: victim was taken by physical force or threatened with bodily harm and then detained for at least 1 hour in an isolated place.

2. Family abduction: victim was taken in violation of a custody order, decree, or other legitimate custodial rights and was concealed or transported outside the state with the intent to prevent return to the rightful caregiver.

3. Victim is a runaway or thrownaway.

   A. *Runaway.* Child voluntarily leaves home at least overnight and is younger than age 14 years or is 15 years or older and stays away for 2 nights.

   B. *Thrownaway.* Child is asked or told to leave home by a parent or other household adult and no adequate alternative-care option is arranged. The child remains out of the home at least overnight.

4. Victim was involuntarily missing, lost, or injured: victim's whereabouts were unknown to the caregiver for at least 1 hour and the caregiver sounded an alarm. The child was unable to contact the caregiver because the child was lost, stranded, injured, or too young to know how to do so.

5. Victim was *caretaker missing*, or missing with a benign explanation in which the child's whereabouts were unknown to the caregiver, causing the caregiver to become alarmed and to try to locate the child. Child was considered reported missing if the caregiver contacts local authorities for the purpose of locating the child.

REFERENCES

Finkelhor D, Hotaling G, Sedlak A. *National Incidence Studies of Missing, Abducted, Runaway, and Thrownaway Children in America* (NISMART). Washington, DC: US Dept of Justice, Office of Justice Programs, Office of Juvenile Justice and Delinquency Prevention; 1990.

Sedlak AJ, Finkelhor D, Hammer H, Schultz DJ. *Second National Incidence Studies of Missing, Abducted, Runaway, and Thrownaway Children in America* (NISMART-2). Washington, DC: US Dept of Justice, Office of Justice Programs, Office of Juvenile Justice and Delinquency Prevention; 2002.

Chapter 17

FAITH-BASED AND RURAL COMMUNITIES

Erika Rivera Ragland, JD
Victor I. Vieth, JD

FAITH-BASED COMMUNITIES

— Both child protection and faith-based communities are charged with protecting children.

1. Faith-based communities tend to interpret their role as keeping families together.

2. Child protective services (CPS) are often seen as breaking families apart.

— Neither group knows enough about the other, resulting in a greater likelihood that the children will not be properly cared for by either.

AREAS OF CONFLICT

— Members of the faith-based community often appear as character witnesses for the accused, so prosecutors and jurors become skeptical of clergy's ability to empathize with, much less protect, victims of child abuse.

1. Clergy may not understand sexual abuse and how easily they can be manipulated. Many clergy lack training in this area or are unprepared to deal with extremely manipulative child abusers.

2. Allegiance to perpetrators may spring from church rules and statutory law. Penitent privilege status can prevent clergy from testifying about inculpatory statements made by criminals. The penitent must give consent for clergypersons to testify on matters disclosed to them in the course of religious duties.

— Clergy may fail to understand or report abuse, often because they do not trust CPS bureaus (Grossoehme, 1998).

— People believe some churches "hide" clergy who are accused of child abuse.

— Many congregations rally around the perpetrator and, in some cases, even blame the victim or the victim's parents. This reflects a long-standing and deeply ingrained belief that God has placed children under the province of parents or other caregivers and that no one, especially not the government, should interfere.

— In cases of child and domestic abuse, some members of the faith community counsel victims to forgive their abusers without requiring accountability under the criminal law and suggest that the doctrine of submission requires endurance of the abuse. Sometimes members fail to speak out.

— Members of the faith-based community often claim scriptural authority for corporal punishment. When this happens, a clash between church and state may occur if the latter deems the discipline to be excessive.

— Many remedial measures taken by the church, such as establishing treatment centers and policies, have proved relatively ineffective and can actually result in returning offenders to their victims. Enforcement of zero-tolerance policies has been met with cynicism, and cases against clergy continue to emerge. Clerical sex offenders share many characteristics with nonclerical offenders (Haywood et al, 1996; Langevin et al, 2000), though clerical offending may be related more to psychosexual adjustment and development issues and less to severe mental disorder (Haywood et al, 1996). The church must report abuse and the CPS and criminal justice systems must treat cases of sexual abuse by clerics the same as cases of sexual abuse by other molesters.

— The CPS community often assumes that members of the faith-based community will be hostile and fails to involve them or even solicit clergy for membership on multidisciplinary teams (MDTs). CPS workers may not keep clergy informed of services that could be accessed to help parents in need.

THE COST
— When faith-based and CPS professionals clash, at least 4 consequences can develop:

1. Children are lost in the church.

2. Victims of domestic violence are lost in the church.

3. Perpetrators are lost in the church. A perpetrator receiving quick forgiveness may assume the sin was not great and offend again.

4. The child's faith needs are lost in the system. Faith issues often arise in cases of child abuse but are ignored.

RECOMMENDATIONS
— Recognize the key role that clergy play in communities. Families in crisis typically do not call social services but do call their pastor, priest, rabbi, or imam. Reach out to local ministerial associations; for example, offer to give a presentation on local efforts to combat child abuse.

— Conduct mandated reporter training for clergy. Separate mandated reporter training for the clergy is appropriate because mandated reporting laws for clergy differ from those for other professionals.

— Develop and use other training materials for the faith-based community. Address the games pedophiles use to obtain access to children in churches and other faith centers.

— Arrange for training from members of the leading faiths in your community. This may include attending various worship services and asking families about their religious practices or beliefs.

— Invite members of the faith-based community to be part of MDTs. This will prepare them to rebut myths and help other team members recognize and respond to faith issues raised by victims.

— Involve members of the faith-based community in prevention programs.

— Teach parishioners how to respond to cases of child abuse and protect their children. Topics can include personal safety and Internet safety for children (**Table 17-1**).

— Take the time to learn about a family's religion and culture and, if possible, work within it.

— Realize that at times disagreements are unavoidable.

— Help the faith-based community establish a system that responds appropriately to the needs of child abuse victims (**Table 17-2**) and domestic violence victims (**Table 17-3**).

Table 17-1. Teaching Personal Safety for Faith-Based Communities

1. Create an atmosphere in which children feel comfortable talking about difficult subjects.

2. Listen to children.

3. Assure children who reveal abuse that they did nothing wrong and that you love them unconditionally.

4. Speak to a pediatrician and a child psychologist about the specifics of the abuse so you can ensure that the child's physical and mental health needs are addressed.

5. Be prepared to respond to the spiritual damage inflicted on the child.

6. Make sure that the church is prepared to address the needs of a child abuse victim. Ask the following questions:

   A. Have the pastors and teachers received training in child abuse issues?

   B. Do the pastors and teachers know the police officers, social workers, and prosecutors who handle child abuse cases in the community?

   C. Are the pastors and teachers familiar with mandated reporting laws and the procedures to be followed in an abuse report?

   D. Does the church library have materials to assist a child or family victimized by abuse?

   E. Does the church school have a good touch/bad touch curriculum?

   F. Do church workers know where to refer a child abuse victim needing professional help?

7. Report the abuse to police.

Table 17-2. Making Congregations Safe for Child Abuse Victims

— Abused children are safe in congregations that understand child abuse can happen anywhere.

— Children are safe in congregations that do not cover up child abuse.

— Abused children are safe in congregations that recognize them as victims and not as sinners.

— Children are safe when congregations do not ostracize those who reveal abuse.

— Children are safer in congregations that give abusers tough love.

Data from Vieth, 1994.

Table 17-3. Making Congregations Safe for Victims of Domestic Violence

— Clergy and congregation must ensure the safety of domestic violence victims.

— Clergy and congregation must care for the spiritual needs of women victimized by violence.

— Congregations must tend to the spiritual and physical needs of children growing up in violent homes.

— Congregations must insist that domestic abusers be held accountable for their sins.

— Congregations should encourage domestic abusers to make themselves right with the law.

— The faith community must resist the temptation to be silent about the sin of domestic violence.

— The faith community must pray that God will guide their efforts to end the assault of spouses and the emotional torture of children.

Data from Vieth, 1996.

Rural Communities

— The naïveté of rural children makes them easier targets for child sexual exploiters than inner-city children (Frank, 2003).

— Characteristics of the victims. See Chapter 2, Victims and Offenders.

— Once rural communities recognize they are not immune from child sexual exploitation (CSE), concrete steps can be taken to protect children from living and dying on the streets.

Approaches

— Use community policing practices.

1. Develop good working relationships with the managers of movie theaters, pool halls, fast food and pizza restaurants, and any other places where teenagers hang out. Ask them to alert the authorities if older persons, especially persons new to the community, start spending time at the facility and speaking to local teenagers.

2. Ask local newspapers and people in the community to immediately contact the authorities if individuals outside the community place an advertisement for teenaged models or other seemingly glamorous jobs outside the town. If the newspapers are uncooperative, explore the possibility of using an administrative subpoena or other police power to investigate the reasonable possibility that such advertisements are a front for CSE.

— Use a community network to identify children at risk.

— Educate children about the dangers of the street.

— Educate parents on how to keep their children safe.

— Closely monitor local strip clubs.

— Develop a network of state and national contacts.

— Address child abuse at the earliest ages.

— Develop forensic interviewing skills applicable to children of all ages.

— Develop investigative abilities appropriate for CSE cases.

— Work closely with social services.

— Publicly advocate for CSE prevention to acquire needed resources.

REFERENCES

Grossoehme DH. Child abuse reporting: clergy perceptions. *Child Abuse Negl.* 1998;7:743-747.

Haywood TW, Kravitz HM, Wasyliw OE, Goldberg J, Cavanaugh JL Jr. Cycle of abuse and psychopathology in cleric and noncleric molesters of children and adolescents. *Child Abuse Negl.* 1996;20: 1233-1243.

Langevin R, Curnoe S, Bain J. A study of clerics who commit sexual offenses: are they different from other sex offenders? *Child Abuse Negl.* 2000;24:535-545.

Vieth VI. Drying their tears: making your congregation safe for child abuse victims. *Northwest Lutheran.* October 1, 1994;81:10.

Vieth VI. When dad hits mom: seven suggestions to make your congregation safe for victims of domestic violence. *Northwest Lutheran.* October 1, 1996;83:10.

Chapter 18

RECOMMENDED ACTIONS

Sharon W. Cooper, MD, FAAP
Richard J. Estes, DSW, ACSW
V. Denise Everett, MD, FAAP
Angelo P. Giardino, MD, PhD, MPH, FAAP
Marcia E. Herman-Giddens, PA, DrPH
Aaron Kipnis, PhD
Ingred Leth, Former Senior Adviser, UNICEF
L. Alvin Malesky, Jr, PhD
Linnea W. Smith, MD

ADVERTISING AND MEDIA INFLUENCES

— The American Academy of Pediatrics (AAP) believes that advertising directed toward children younger than 8 years is inherently deceptive and exploitive.

— Until the age of 5 years, children cannot differentiate between commercials and programming. Only when they reach age 8 years do children realize advertisements exist to sell products.

— Juveniles live in a culture where advertising sets no clear boundary between commercial messages or imagery and the real world.

— Parents are often overwhelmed and undermined when trying to monitor and restrict children's access to sexually explicit or exploitive media.

1. The average child aged 8 to 18 years spends 6 hours, 43 minutes per day with media.

2. Those aged 9 to 17 years use the Internet 4 days a week, averaging 2 hours online at a time.

3. By high school graduation, young people will have watched 15 000 hours of television but spent only 12 000 hours in school.

4. The average American adolescent views almost 14 000 sexual references per year; only 165 deal with birth control, abstinence, self-control, risk of pregnancy, or sexually transmitted diseases.

5. 56% of all television programs contain sexual content.

6. Teenagers rank the media as a source of sexual information second only to school sex education.

— Advertising that sexually exploits children appears in mainstream magazines with a wide readership throughout society.

— Symbols of pain, torture, and sadomasochism are glamorized in mainstream advertising, implying that subordination and suffering can produce sexual gratification.

— Most video games, music, and movies, including those with R ratings (children younger than 17 years must be accompanied by a parent or guardian to enter), are promoted to children.

— Children's media consumption, especially of violent, gender-stereotyped, sexually explicit, or drug- and alcohol-influenced media, skews their world view with respect to frequency of sexual activity, number of sexual partners, and sexual norms. Consumption correlates with increased high-risk behavior and accelerates the onset of sexual activity.

— Much media attention is focused on a female body type considerably below normal body weight.

CHILDREN'S ADVERTISING REVIEW UNIT

— Children's Advertising Review Unit promotes responsible advertising to children (those younger than 12 years) and responds to public concerns.

— 7 principles underlie the unit's guidelines. Specifically, advertisers:

1. Should consider the level of knowledge, sophistication, and maturity of their audience.

2. Should not exploit children's imaginative quality.

3. Should not advertise or promote directly to children products and content inappropriate for their use.

4. Must communicate appropriate information truthfully, accurately, and in language understandable to young children, recognizing that children may learn practices that can affect their health and well-being.

5. Are urged to develop advertising that addresses positive and beneficial social behavior.

6. Should incorporate minority and other groups and present positive and prosocial roles and role models.

7. Must contribute constructively to the parent–child relationship, recognizing that parents have the primary responsibility to guide children.

LET KIDS BE KIDS

— Committee on Child Abuse & Neglect of the North Carolina Pediatric Society launched Let Kids Be Kids as a campaign against the sexual exploitation of children in advertising.

— It is designed to discourage companies from using advertising that portrays children as sexual objects.

— The North Carolina Pediatric Society produces brochures, video-tapes, and other promotional material that describes the problem. Brochure content emphasizes that physicians, parents, and others interested in this issue can do the following:

1. Write or call advertisers who sexually exploit children in their advertisements.

2. Educate colleagues about the problem.

3. Talk to children if they are exposed to these advertisements to address any resulting confusion.

4. Discourage companies or businesses from advertising in this manner.

5. Support advertisers using healthy, nonsexual, and age-appropriate themes and let them know of your support.

6. Promote media literacy courses that include sexuality issues in schools.

— The campaign targets:

1. Advertisements featuring children wearing provocative clothing, appearing in suggestive poses, or touching private parts

2. Advertisements featuring adult models acting sexually desirable while they are made to look like children

— The resulting national effort was supported by AAP.

DADS AND DAUGHTERS

— National nonprofit membership group for fathers and daughters.

— Urges all teen magazines to demand that advertisers stop glorifying unhealthy body images.

PEDIATRICIANS

— The AAP leads in recognizing the role of mass media in child health and development, reviewing research, advocating policy, and developing and implementing professional and public education campaigns.

— Have the unique position of both proximity and a commitment to the welfare of children.

— The AAP and the American Association of Child and Adolescent Psychiatrists recommend that pediatricians, child psychiatrists, and child health professionals add a simple media history to the health profile taken during routine office visits (Arehart-Treichel, 2001; Wingood et al, 2001).

1. If the evaluation reveals heavy media use, suggest healthy alternatives and evaluate for aggressive behavior, fears, or sleep disturbances.

2. Use brochures suggesting ways to guide families toward positive media uses, establish a healthy "media diet" with limits and

balance, and carry out critical discussions of what children read and watch.

3. Explore the sexual content of media preferences to expose misinformation and provide an opportunity to discuss sexuality issues.

— Provide only socially responsible, child-positive magazines, periodicals, and other media choices to patients in outpatient waiting rooms and inpatient settings.

— Prescreen print media, videotapes, and videogames for violent and/or sexually explicit content.

— Review editorial content as well as advertising images and messages.

— Encourage and facilitate professional organizations and child advocacy groups to establish content guidelines for popular media available in child/adolescent healthcare settings.

— Obtain child-friendly instructional materials to help them develop media literacy skills as well as material to help educate parents.

— Develop outreach programs to increase awareness and encourage the use of conduct codes in modeling agencies and professional photography groups.

— Lobby to establish position statements on the responsible portrayal of children in advertising and guidelines to prevent harming children working in commercial media.

— Emphasize profitability as well as social responsibility in the business community.

— Encourage the AAP to form a committee to study how children and adolescents can be harmed in the media and whether to work to pass legislation to raise the minimum age for models in sexually explicit media to 21 years.

— Encourage people to:

1. Advocate for stricter limits on the amount of advertising on children's television.

2. Hold corporations and businesses accountable by not buying their products.

3. Praise appropriate advertising and patronize responsible businesses.

4. Suggest parents spend their dollars on consumer goods that do not exploit children with harmful products or advertising.

5. Write offending companies letters of thoughtful concern and motivate other colleagues and parents to write. Encourage similar projects for older children and adolescents as individuals and groups.

6. Write, phone, or e-mail local newspapers and radio and television stations that run irresponsible advertisements.

7. Encourage parents to teach media literacy and ask their children's schools to do the same. Ask leaders at the neighborhood school if they have a media literacy program that addresses advertising and sexuality; if not, volunteer to serve on a committee to develop needed programs.

8. Help to raise public awareness by suggesting and supporting school, civic group, and church programs as well as by developing and attending workshops on advertising, media, and sexuality.

9. Support media groups that promote more balanced, realistic, age-appropriate, and diverse portrayals of girls, boys, men, and women in advertising.

10. Encourage professional associations and child advocacy organizations to develop position statements on the nonexploitive use of children in advertising and the targeting of children by advertisers.

11. Build coalitions with other professional and community groups, including early childhood professions and parent-teacher organizations, education and public health departments, and state attorneys general.

— Help parents raise media-resilient children by taking the following steps:

1. Remind parents that advertising represents commercial speech, not free speech, and the Federal Trade Commission is empowered to ban unfair or deceptive ads.

2. Encourage them to expect the media to take responsibility for its actions and play a role in the public health of society.

3. Advise them to limit children's access and exposure to media, especially when young, and to establish good media habits early.

4. Encourage them to discuss media with their children.

5. Reinforce the fact that though children may protest and disagree, they will remember what was said and may not experience the images or messages in the same way again.

6. Brainstorm ways for parents to more effectively share about media experience and impact, and establish an open and ongoing dialogue with their children.

7. Support those who may feel devalued and stigmatized for being critical of the powerfully pervasive and youth-focused popular culture.

8. Encourage parents to mute commercial breaks on the television or to at least point out marketing techniques.

— The most important action is to learn more and to be able to tell the difference between what is educational, age-appropriate, developmentally appropriate, and healthy, and what is dehumanizing and exploitive.

REINTEGRATION

— Ideally, children who have been trafficked and exploited should return to their families, but the solution is not that simple.

— Often rehabilitation in the community where the children are found is preferable.

— The major obstacle is ostracism.

INTERNATIONAL CONVENTIONS/PROTOCOLS

Commit governments to protect children from all forms of physical or mental violence, including sexual abuse.

PREVENTIVE MEASURES

— Sexual abuse and exploitation are less frequent in countries with:

1. A tradition of education for girls and boys.

2. Free access to sex education.

3. A high level of social control in the community.

4. Equality between genders.

5. Political and economic stability.

6. A high level of social and healthcare services.

7. Efficient legislation regarding child protection.

8. Efficient legislation to prosecute perpetrators.

9. Efficient law enforcement.

10. Cultural mainstream emphasizing the principles supporting children's rights.

FOSTER CARE ISSUES

— Foster children come most often from young family systems that fail to thrive; more than half a million US children will be in government-run foster care homes each year.

— Although the system was designed to provide temporary care for abused, abandoned, and neglected children, many of those committed remain in state custody for years.

— Girls are highly favored over boys for adoption, so boys tend to remain longer.

— Many youths are simply warehoused in understaffed environments until they reach the age of 18 years (Courtney, 1998).

MEASURES TO REDUCE CHILD ABUSE INCIDENCE

— Provide better support for impoverished parents to achieve economic self-sufficiency and education, understanding that economic stress alone can contribute to a higher incidence of child abuse and neglect.

— When violence occurs in a home, ensure that parents and caregivers are mandated to anger management programs and drug and alcohol treatment programs where applicable.

— Dedicate more public resources to protecting foster children, knowing they do not have the political power to lobby on their own behalf.

— Support programs to assist fathers in developing the emotional, technical, and financial capacity to be positively involved in their children's lives.

— Initiate aggressive adoption campaigns, including economic incentives and professional support networks, for all US children currently left in institutions.

— Require high schools and marriage license grantors to provide all teenagers and newlyweds with parenting instruction.

— Require all divorcing couples with children to attend joint childcare planning before granting a divorce.

— Implore teachers, doctors, coaches, counselors, clergy members, parents, and neighbors to speak directly to children who appear abused or to contact authorities. Whenever it is safe to do so, talk to adults who are abusing their children in public.

— Abolish the notion that any adult should be allowed to strike any child, anywhere, for any reason.

— Support helplines and hotlines for those individuals who are contemplating committing a sexual offense against children but are seeking prevention assistance (such as that provided by Stop It Now).

— Empower juvenile bystanders in universal public awareness campaigns specific to sexual exploitation, a method that has already been implemented and shown to be successful in drinking and driving campaigns.

— Encourage faith communities to include child abuse in their teaching and outreach, particularly in rural communities.

MEASURES TO REDUCE CHILD HOMELESSNESS

— Provide shelters that have the educational, medical, and vocational support needed to help homeless youths stay off the streets.

— Challenge the biases that bar homeless boys and young men access to shelters.

— Train social workers on how to reach out to homeless young men on the streets where they live.

— Ensure that all youths leaving foster care, juvenile institutions, or jails have the resources they need to transition from institutional to independent living.

— Implement primary prevention, treatment, and diversion programs, wherever possible, to keep children from becoming homeless.

— Support mentoring programs that connect children at risk with caring, capable, and responsible adults.

— Increase entry-level employment opportunities for youths in jobs with upward mobility and a living wage.

RECOMMENDATIONS FOR REHABILITATION PROGRAMS (MILLER, 1998)

— Move youthful offenders out of remote, isolated institutions into secured environments near populations that can provide educational and social services, community volunteer programs, and regular interactions with family members, as appropriate.

— Reduce caseloads of probation officers so they can provide intensive supervision and integrated support services for youths returning to the community.

— Establish citizen oversight of locked institutions (similar to police review boards) to ensure zero tolerance toward abuse and neglect of children.

— End solitary confinement and corporal punishment in all juvenile institutions.

— Provide juvenile mental patients rights against involuntary commitment and medication equal to those granted adults.

— Increase public awareness about how expanded criminalizing and pathologizing of young male behavior is skyrocketing the rates of hospitalizations and incarcerations.

— Provide substance abuse treatment, therapy, education, parenting education, and literacy and vocational training in all locked juvenile facilities to help break the generational cycles of poverty and violence.

— Enact zero tolerance toward rape, sexual slavery, and forced prostitution of youths in prisons.

— Create more voluntary community treatment centers, staffed with professionals trained to help youths at risk, that can stand between troubled boys and locked institutions.

— Once the centers are established, eliminate juvenile halls and prisons except for the minority of incarcerated youths who are a proven threat to public safety.

RECOMMENDATIONS FOR EVALUATING AND TREATING INTERNET-RELATED SEX OFFENDERS

— The goal is to enable offenders to identify situations that place them at risk to reoffend (Nelson & Jackson, 1989).

1. Internet usage is a high-risk activity to be avoided.

2. Professionals involved in the treatment and/or community monitoring of Internet sex offenders should prohibit Internet usage or at least closely monitor the offender's online activity.

— Clinical recommendation: Offenders should focus on developing and strengthening "real-life" prosocial adult relationships instead of spending excessive time online.

1. Ensuring complete compliance with Internet restriction for all

offenders is virtually impossible, but take steps to minimize the possibility of deviant or illegal Internet use.

  A. Encourage Internet offenders employed in the computer/ Internet fields to pursue employment opportunities where they are not required to work extensively with computers or on the Internet.

  B. Actively monitor online activity.

  C. Do not allow Internet offenders to have Internet access in their homes. If the presence of other family members or roommates makes this suggestion unrealistic, closely monitor the offender to ensure the Internet is not misused.

2. Provide specialized training for probation and parole officers focusing on computer usage and the Internet to assist them in monitoring offenders.

— Educate forensic evaluators and treatment providers involved with Internet-related sex offender cases about Internet technology.

1. Ensure they are familiar with its unique aspects.

2. Equip evaluators to actively monitor newsgroups containing information related to their case (McGrath & Casey, 2002).

3. Recognize that more research is needed.

REFERENCES

Arehart-Treichel J. Psychiatrist helps pediatricians develop antiviolence statement. *Psychiatr News*. 2001;36(24):14.

Courtney M. *Foster Facts*. Madison, Wis: Irving Piliavin School of Social Work, University of Wisconsin; 1998.

McGrath MG, Casey E. Forensic psychiatry and the Internet: practical perspectives on sexual predators and obsessional harassers in cyber-space. *J Am Acad Psychiatry Law*. 2002;30(1):81-94.

Miller J. *Last One Over the Wall*. 2nd ed. Columbus, Ohio: Ohio State University Press; 1998.

Nelson C, Jackson P. High-risk recognition: the cognitive-behavioral chain. In: Laws DR, ed. *Relapse Prevention With Sex Offenders*. New York, NY: The Guilford Press; 1989:167-177.

Wingood GM, DiClemente FJ, Harrington K, Davies S, Hook EW, Oh MK. Exposure to X-rated movies and adolescents' sexual and contraceptive-related attitudes and behaviors. *Pediatrics*. 2001;107: 1116-1119.

INDEX

A

E

G

Gammahydroxybutyrate (GHB), usage/withdrawal (symptoms), 120t
Gasoline, usage/withdrawal (symptoms), 120t
Gateway, 205, 220
Gender, identification/analysis, 174-175
Generic top-level domain (gTLD), definition, 220
Genital injuries, 147
    assessment, 121-125
        position, 121-123
Genital trauma, differential diagnosis, 139-141
Genitalia, normal appearance, 136-141
GHB. *See* Gammahydroxybutyrate
Girls, genitalia (normal appearance), 137-139
Global travelers, definition, 73
Glue, usage/withdrawal (symptoms), 120t
Gonorrhea, 128
    prophylactic treatment, 133t, 134t
Good faith exception, 251-252
Good practice, principles. *See* Prostituted children
Governmental organizations (GOs), 104-105
Graphical image file, bit-stream copy, 261
Grooming, 34-35
   steps. *See* Victims
Group sessions, usage, 282
gTLD. *See* Generic top-level domain
Guardian ad litem, role, 243t
Guides, 38t
Guilt, shame (contrast), 162

H

Habituation, definition, 72
Hacker/intrusion defenses, defeating, 267
Hallucinogens, usage/withdrawal (symptoms), 119t-120t
Hare Psychopathy Checklist, 153
Header, 220
HEADSS. *See* Home, Education/employment, Activity, Drugs, Sexuality,
    Suicide/depression screen
Healing groups, stages, 273-274
Healthcare
   professionals, interaction, 63-64
   settings. *See* Prostituted children

O

P

Y

Z

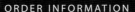
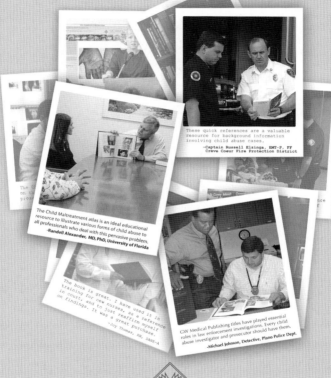

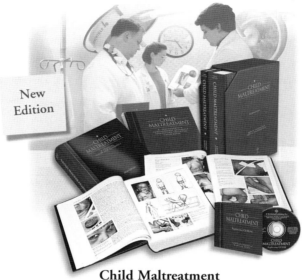

Quickly find digital images to help identify physical abuse

The *Child Maltreatment Supplementary CD-ROM* contains 300 full-color images with detailed case studies from field experts. All of the images are from our *Child Maltreatment Photographic Reference* and illustrate a diverse and comprehensive range of maltreatment and abuse circumstances. With the addition of a new slide presentation on physical abuse, this resource perfectly complements the 2-volume set for training presentations or self-study.

Contents

To order call toll-free **1-800-600-0330**

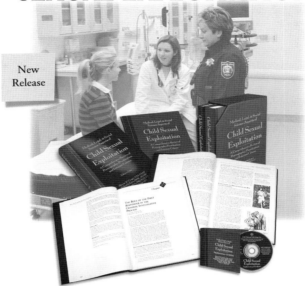

Addressing problems that arise from our global world, these books will be the standard for *law enforcement, medical, forensic, legal,* and *social science* professionals in the 21st century, empowering them to help stop this type of abuse.

Learn techniques used by lawbreakers in a multimedia environment

The *Child Sexual Exploitation Supplementary CD-ROM* is a researcher's companion to the 2-volume set. Users can learn how photos are circulated on the Internet and to spot digitally altered images. Users may also browse the extensive collection of more than 100 articles and government documents from the United States and abroad, assemble a collection of best practices from federal and local agencies, or create their own training curriculum using slide shows and case studies of sexual maturation, taxonomy of pornography, and sexually transmitted diseases.

Contents

To order call toll-free **1-800-600-0330**

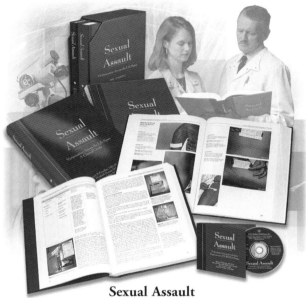

The *Sexual Assault Color Atlas* contains actual case studies from experts in the field, including more than 1400 high-quality clinical photos of sexually transmitted diseases, injuries in progressive stages of healing, and comparisons of injuries in multiple age groups. The atlas has special sections on victims with disabilities, assault during incarceration, cases involving DNA collection and analysis, and steps for prosecution.

The value of these two references cannot be overstated. Used together, they will aid professionals in dealing with sexual assault victims and lead the way to better evaluation and interpretation of their injuries.

Document and investigate sexual assault with the digital image library

The *Sexual Assault Supplementary CD-ROM* contains 130 full-color images with detailed case studies, all taken from the *Sexual Assault Color Atlas*, reflecting the findings that are most characteristic of the various age groups. The CD-ROM is a perfect complement to the 2-volume set, whether for training presentations or self-study.

Contents

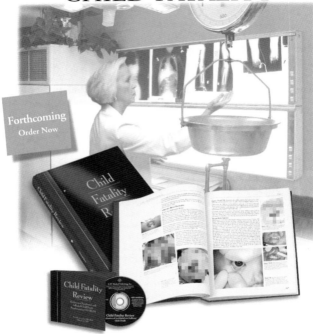

Case studies illustrate abusive and accidental forms of death, including neglect, SIDS, suicide, burning, drowning, and infectious diseases. This text is a powerful tool for all members of a child fatality review team and can guide anyone trying to form a new team.

While this illustrated text is an excellent tool for anyone who works on or with child fatality review teams, it is also an asset in the education arena. This reference is a valuable teaching tool in university social work classes or law enforcement teaching facilities.

Conveniently create presentations and test abilities with the CD-ROM

The *Child Fatality Review Supplementary CD-ROM* provides additional information to all professionals on these teams and allows members to test their abilities in reviewing difficult cases. It is a perfect complement to the text, whether for training presentations or self study.

Contents*

† page and image counts are approximate.

* contents are subject to change

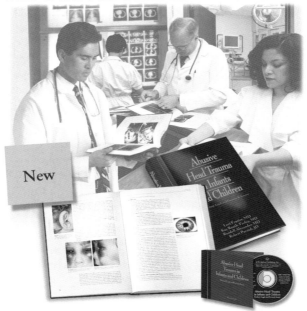

More than 600 clinical photos, case studies, and multidisciplinary analyses illustrate inflicted head injuries. Discussions of shaken baby syndrome, shaken impact syndrome, differential diagnoses, forensic analyses, autopsies, prosecutorial issues, long-term care of survivors, and the role of social services are featured.

This single-volume edition combines the best clinical writing with high-quality photographic content—a wealth of knowledge bound in one concise edition.

Show the reality of shaken baby syndrome with 3-D animations

The *Abusive Head Trauma Supplementary CD-ROM* uses 3-D images and animation developed from actual forensic analysis of victimized children to depict how head injuries occur. This product is valuable for explaining the complex biomechanics of abusive head injury to investigators, and mandated reporters in an easy-to-understand format. Distinguish shaken baby syndrome from other types of head trauma with exacting animations developed by an esteemed pathologist.

Contents

TRAINING MATERIALS

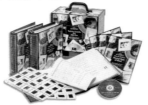

Child Maltreatment:
Training Module and Visuals

Angelo P. Giardino, MD, PhD, FAAP; James A. Monteleone, MD

34 contributors

Training Module and Visuals *ISBN 1-878060-29-5* $469.95
Additional $125 to order images in both CD-ROM and 35-mm format

Train anyone to identify, interpret, and report child abuse and neglect

Written by 34 leading experts in various areas of child maltreatment, these training modules include a CD-ROM with 392 full-color images; three 3-ring binders, each with approximately 225 pages and 36 lessons; 9 student workbooks; and 16 transparency acetate overheads.

This package is customizable for anyone who trains or teaches others how to *identify, interpret,* and *report* child abuse, including *law enforcement officers, attorneys, medical professionals, prehospital personnel, mental health professionals, social workers,* and *teachers.*

Contents

SEXUAL ASSAULT
Quick Reference

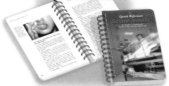

Sexual Assault Quick Reference
For Health Care, Social Service, and Law Enforcement Professionals

Angelo P. Giardino, MD, PhD, FAAP; Elizabeth M. Datner, MD;
Janice B. Asher, MD; Barbara W. Girardin, RN, PhD;
Diana K. Faugno, RN, BSN, CPN, FAAFS, SANE-A; Mary J. Spencer, MD

560 pages, 150 images, 69 contributors

Sexual Assault Quick Reference *ISBN 1-878060-38-4* $49.95

Quickly access information about sexual assault while on the front line

The *Sexual Assault Quick Reference* is an invaluable resource and field guide in a convenient pocket-sized format providing easy access to information for medical, forensic, and law enforcement investigations of sexual assault. Topics covered include the roles of multi-disciplinary teams, abusive and nonabusive variants, physical and forensic evaluation procedures, STDs, domestic violence, DNA collection and testing, disabled victims, and preparing for prosecution.

This text illustrates the problems of sexual assault and abuse through the eyes of many professionals, and the knowledge shared supplies others with the power to intervene. People in any related area can use this information to become empowered participants whose effective interventions help prevent sexual assault and care for its victims. Data are current, accurate, and specific to sexual assault, and the processes of detecting sexual assault, caring for victims, and prosecuting lawbreakers are thoroughly explained.

Contents

1. Principle of Sexual Assault at Any Age
2. Anogenital Anatomy
3. Physical Evaluation of Children
4. Forensic Evaluation of Children
5. Differential Diagnosis
6. Evaluations in Special Situations
7. Multidisciplinary Teamwork Issues
8. Documentation and Reporting
9. Physical Evaluation of Adolescents and Adults

10. Forensic Evaluation of Adolescents and Adults
11. Sexually Transmitted Diseases and Pregnancy
12. Violence and Rape Issues
13. Special Settings
14. Psychological and Social Supports
15. Caregiver Issues
16. Legal Issues, Investigation, and Prosecution

To order call toll-free **1-800-600-0330**

CHILD ABUSE
Quick Reference

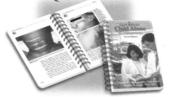

Child Abuse Quick Reference
For Health Care, Social Service, and Law Enforcement Professionals
Second Edition

Angelo P. Giardino, MD, PhD, MPH, FAAP
Randell Alexander, MD, PhD, FAAP

448 pages, 155 images, 93 contributors

Child Abuse Quick Reference Second Edition *ISBN 1-878060-60-0* $46.95

Quickly and easily access information about medical aspects of child abuse when and where it is needed

For medical, social service, law enforcement, and legal professionals working with children, the most essential information concerning child maltreatment identification and diagnosis can be found in this convenient reference. The essential information is condensed here in the form of bulleted outlines, lists, tables, and high-quality clinical photos.

The chapters address the most common types of child abuse as well as uncommon but possible causes such as cultural or religious practices that often look like abuse. The format is arranged to identify an issue, describe methods of assessment and treatment, point out essentials of investigation and prosecution, and summarize education and prevention strategies. Frontline professionals in hospitals, clinics, law enforcement agencies, and many other organizations often confront allegations of child abuse. This reference is designed to help professionals rapidly access the information they need to tackle child abuse.

Contents

To order or for more information, visit **www.gwmedical.com**

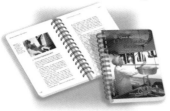
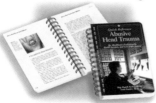

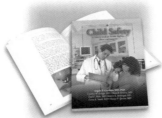
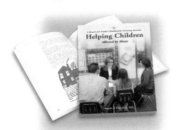